"Roger has filled a yawning gap in our knowled[ge of] our community. Using a multitude of sources [...] doctors, nurses and others who have served this [...] as human beings."

Dr Ken Sneath, Dar[...]

"A magnificent effort which I thoroughly enjoyed reading. I am aware of only one other practice which can trace its history as far back as this."

Dr Mike Muncaster, Independent Lecturer on the History of Medicine.

"A very interesting read and a lovely insight into the history of the practice. Something for future generations to refer to."

Elish Millard, vice-chair of the Patients' Forum.

"In medicine we learn the most from patient narratives, their stories. Here we have the doctors' stories illuminating and humanising General Practice in our community."

Dr Alex Connan.

"A great read, with a whole lot of historical facts that build the story of 'medical' Huntingdon and Godmanchester."

Richard Pumphrey, Patients' Forum.

"A fascinating history of the practice over the past 200 years."

Dr Richard Weyell, retired GP with the Charles Hicks Practice.

"Roger has produced a well-researched and fascinating history of our local medical practice, full of interesting social history and details of the lives of those involved. I am glad to be living today and not 200 years ago when comparing medical provision then and now! We have much to be thankful for."

Dorne Burdett, local resident.

"A thoroughly researched and engaging account of the development of GP services in Godmanchester and Huntingdon with anecdotes that make the actors come alive. I learned a lot and enjoyed reading it. I am sure it will be appreciated by many."

Dr Martin Becker, retired consultant paediatrician, Hinchingbrooke Hospital.

"A fascinating read. It was lovely to read the history of the surgery and the GPs."

Irena Hall, receptionist at the Charles Hicks Practice.

"Amazing how little the early doctors had to treat patients. Surgery with very little anaesthetic and few medicines. No wonder they had to rely so heavily on opiates!"

Rosemary Smith, Patients' Forum.

"Roger's excellent research on the history and development of the surgeries of Huntingdon and Godmanchester is a fascinating narration of the medical history of our region and a welcome nod to our memories of the wonderful doctors, nurses and surgery staff who have selflessly given their time, knowledge and at times friendship over the years. For 47 years, they have looked after and cared for us during the day and in the middle of the night. It is a pleasure to be reminded of all of them. It is also very interesting to see the development of medicine and care, as time has passed. Thank you, Roger, for a good read, for refreshing my memory and reminding me of how lucky we are to have such a dedicated medical team taking care of us."

Macha Pumphrey, Patients' Forum.

In Sickness and in Health
The story of the Charles Hicks Practice

In Sickness and in Health

The story of the Charles Hicks Practice

Roger Merritt

With a Foreword by
Dr Ken Sneath

This publication has been made possible by a grant from the
Goodliff Fund of the Huntingdonshire Local History Society

Published by the Patients' Forum of the Hicks Group Practice.

Email: patientsforum.CHS@gmail.com

First published in Great Britain in 2024

Copyright © Patients' Forum 2024

Copyright text © Roger Merritt 2024

The right of Roger Merritt to be identified as the author of this work has been asserted by him in accordance with the Copyright, Designs and Patents Act 1988.

No part of this publication may be reproduced by any means, stored in a retrieval system, distributed or transmitted in any form by electronic, mechanical, recording or otherwise, without the permission of the Patients' Forum and the copyright owner.

British Library Cataloguing-in-Publication data.
A CIP record of this title is available from the British Library.

Paperback ISBN – 978-1-916838-82-6

Cover design and page design by Kevin Moore.
Printed in Great Britain by Biddles Books Ltd, Kings Lynn.

Front cover images, clockwise from top left: Group of doctors including Herbert Lucas, at Huntingdon County Hospital in the 1890s (courtesy Cambridgeshire archives), Charles Hicks and his name plate, Nelson Hicks, Bosworth House, a medical bag belonging to Herbert Lucas, and Hicks Group doctors at the opening of the Godmanchester Roman Gate surgery (all Hicks Group archive), the Roman Gate surgery (Patients' Forum), a Red Cross nurse in WW1 (Hicks Group archive), Jim Rushton (courtesy Hunts Post), Michael Foster (courtesy Cambridgeshire archives), a 19th century surgeons set (courtesy the Norris Museum).

Back cover image: the plaque at the centre of a painting at the Roman Gate surgery (Patients' Forum).

This book is dedicated to the memory of Sandra (Sandy) Ferrelly. Sandy co-founded the Patients' Forum at the Charles Hicks Practice in 2009 and admirably chaired the group for most of the next 10 years. "She was a very good friend to the Practice, and we were all very grateful to her." (Dr Whitton)

Sandy's career was spent working for the NHS at St Thomas' Hospital in London. On her retirement to Godmanchester she dedicated her knowledge and expertise to support various voluntary groups in the community, of which the Patients' Forum was fortunate to be one.

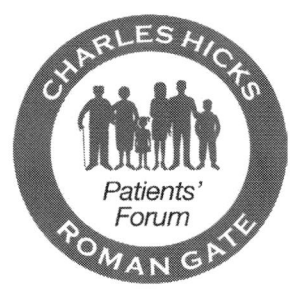

"Let us therefore praise famous men by all means but not forget the work of the man in the field of 100 years ago, who had to cope in 90% of cases with inadequate or no facilities and little but his sound common sense and the milk of human kindness to guide him."

    Charles Hicks in a letter to his son Nelson Hicks, on handing over his Practice in 1948.

"Illness is neither an indulgence for which people should have to pay, nor an offence for which they should be penalised, but a misfortune, the cost of which should be shared by the community."

    Nye Bevan on the founding of the NHS in 1948.

"We continue to be at the forefront of innovation, whilst maintaining a responsive, caring service for our patients. The future will no doubt throw further challenges at us, but we are ready to face them."

    Dr Carolyn Smithson, partner in the Hicks Group Practice in 2024.

Table of Contents

Acknowledgements and permissions			xi
Abbreviations			xiii
Foreword			1
Introduction			3
Chapter 1	Early medical practitioners	(1793–1803)	5
Chapter 2	Jonah Wilson	(1809–1848)	11
Chapter 3	Michael Foster	(1833–1876)	17
Chapter 4	Herbert Lucas	(1863–1919)	27
Chapter 5	Charles Hicks	(1910–1948)	37
Chapter 6	Nelson Hicks	(1948–1973)	55
Chapter 7	Jim Rushton	(1965–1995)	65
Chapter 8	Up to the present day	(1995–2024)	77
Appendix 1	Timelines		87
Appendix 2	Women and Healthcare		91
Appendix 3	One patient's story		95
References			97
Index of Names			107
General Index			109

Acknowledgements

Grateful thanks are due to:

Expert readers who commented on the full text: Dr Richard Weyell, Dr Alex Connan, Dr Mike Muncaster and Dr Martin Becker. Other readers included Patients' Forum members, Elish Millard, Rosemary Smith and Richard and Macha Pumphrey, also Roy Millard, Josephine Becker, Dorne Burdett, Pam Sneath and Denise Merritt-Kwan.

Many people from the Hicks Group Practice past and present, have supported this project. From the current staff Dr Ian Sweetenham and Dr Carolyn Smithson, Lisa Harrison and Irena Hall all contributed in-person and online interviews, together with photographs and access to items from the archives at the Practice. Past staff interviewees with reminiscences and photographs have included Dr Mike Whitton, Dr Keith Stewart, Sharon Gray, Wendy Stukins, Lesley Wood and Jean Huff.

We wanted the reminiscences of many patients over the years to contribute to the project. Patient interviewees have brought the project to life; they include John and Biz Thackray, Verna Hayes, Danny Reid and Chis Selym. Stories of the Charles Hicks and other practices in Godmanchester and Huntingdon were contributed though lively Facebook discussions on *'Old Codgers and Codgesses of Godmanchester'* and *'History of Huntingdon High Street'*. Many thanks to all who posted on those sites, some of whose voices are represented in the final text. My apologies to anyone who I have missed.

Other people who have contributed with research suggestions and archives access are Philip Saunders of Huntingdon History Society, along with Sue Sampson and the fantastic team at the Huntingdon Library archives. Thanks also to Lesley Akeroyd at the Norris Museum in St Ives and Liz Davies, local historian. David Stokes at Godmanchester Porch Museum supported the project throughout.

Alan Hooker and Stephen Spencer have helped with photographs and print advice. Colin Hyams and Kevin Moore have contributed their invaluable professional insights and cover and page design expertise.

Last, but not least, Ken Sneath has been my mentor throughout the project with advice on local history research, referencing, indexing and much more beside. Ken really did go 'above and beyond'. This project could not have happened without him. Any mistakes remaining in the text are entirely my own.

Thanks also to the committee of the Patients' Forum for their commitment and support for this project throughout the past year.

The financial contribution from the Goodliff Fund was welcome and the Patients' Forum is very grateful. All proceeds from the sales of this book will go to the Patients' Forum funds for purchase of equipment and amenities to enhance the patient experience at the Charles Hicks Practice.

Finally, to Judith, without whom none of this would have been possible. My love and grateful thanks as ever.

Copyright

Owners of copyright are identified beneath each illustration or photograph in the text. Grateful thanks are due to the following:

The Wellcome collection for works made available under Public Domain Mark or Attribution 4.0 International Licence. Pages 5, 6, 7, 9, 10, 12, 13, 14, 18, 23, 24, 26, 30, 34, 38, 45, 56.

The Hicks Group archives. Pages 28, 31, 39, 40, 43, 44, 49, 50, 51, 53, 54, 55, 57, 58, 59, 62, 63, 64, 68, 69, 71, 72, 74, 75, 77, 78, 79, 81, 83, 91, 93.

Cambridgeshire Archives. Pages 8, 15, 20, 29, 33, 35, 41, 42, 44, 46, 48, 51, 60.

Patients' Forum archives. Pages 35, 70, 72, 73, 76, 80, 82, 84, 86, 93, 95.

The Norris Museum of St Ives. Pages 20, 24.

The Thackray Museum of Medicine. Pages 12, 22.

The Cambridge Community Archive Network. Pages 19, 21.

Dr Alex Connan. Pages 47, 92.

Verna Hayes. Pages 59, 61.

The Hunts Post. Page 65.

Les Williams. Page 67.

Every effort has been made to contact copyright holders. The publishers will be pleased to rectify any omission in future editions.

ABBREVIATIONS

ARRS	Additional Roles Reimbursement Scheme
BA	Batchelor of Arts
BMA	British Medical Association
CCG	Clinical Commissioning Group
CM	Certified Midwife
CQC	Care Quality Commission
ENT	Ear, Nose and Throat
FRCS	Fellow of Royal College of Surgeons
FRS	Fellow of the Royal Society
GMC	General Medical Council
GP	General Practitioner
ICB	Integrated Care Board
ICP	Integrated Care Partnership
KCB	Knight Commander of the order of the Bath
LRCP	Licentiate of College of Physicians
LRCS	Licentiate of College of Surgeons
LSA	Licentiate of Society of Apothecaries
MAGPAS	Mid Anglia General Practitioner Accident Service
MB	Batchelor of Medicine and Surgery
MD	Doctor of Medicine (higher research degree)
MO	Medical Officer
MOH	Medical Officer of Health
MP	Member of Parliament
MRCP	Member of Royal College of Physicians
MRCS	Member of Royal College of Surgeons
NHSE	National Health Service England
NICE	National Institute for Health and Care Excellence
PCN	Primary Care Network
PCT	Primary Care Trust
PHC	Primary Health Care
PMS	Personal Medical Services

PPG	Patient Participation Group
QOF	Quality and Outcomes Framework
RAMC	Royal Army Medical Corps
RCN	Royal College of Nursing
VMH	Victoria Medal of Honour

Foreword

I am delighted to be asked to contribute the foreword to this excellent book by Roger Merritt. The story of healthcare in Godmanchester and Huntingdon had very humble beginnings 200 years ago and the medical advances in the intervening centuries would have astounded those early pioneers.

Roger is the current Chairman of the Patients' Forum, and he has developed a keen interest in the history of healthcare in this area. With energy and commitment, he has charted the enormous strides in treatment in the face of threats to health, which have included the epidemics of smallpox, cholera, 'Spanish Flu' and most recently COVID. Using a multitude of sources he has uncovered the lives of the doctors, nurses and others who have served this area. He has also revealed them as human beings. Who knew that Dr Nelson Hicks used his own childhood teddy bear to help his youngest patients identify where they were hurting?

A number of volumes on Godmanchester's fascinating history have been produced since the turn of the century, from Tim Malim and Michael Green on the town's archaeology, my books on Godmanchester's 800-year history including its church, the pubs and its transport and Roger Leivers on the Second World War. But none of us have attempted a history of healthcare. Roger has admirably filled this yawning gap in our knowledge, and I have no hesitation in commending it to the people of the town.

Dr Ken Sneath
Darwin College
University of Cambridge

INTRODUCTION

This book began with a visit to the Roman Gate surgery in Godmanchester in 2022. How many readers have looked up in the entrance lobby when visiting the surgery? If you have, you will have seen a painting by Roy Larcombe over the door. It shows on one side the previous surgery at Old Court Hall, and on the other side the new Roman Gate surgery before the recent extension. At the centre of the painting is this plaque:

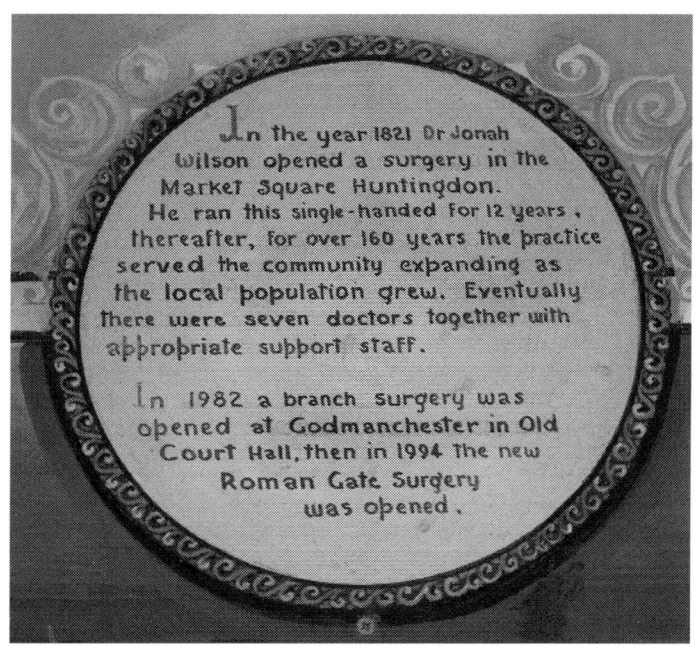

Reading that date of 1821 made me realise that the 200-year anniversary of the Practice had fallen in the middle of the COVID pandemic and had therefore been understandably overlooked. This raised several questions which this book seeks to answer:

- How did staff at the Charles Hicks Practice cope during the COVID pandemic and what challenges remain today?
- What other sicknesses and diseases have impacted on the residents of Huntingdon and Godmanchester over the years? What caused them, and how were they treated?
- Who was Charles Hicks and who else has provided local medical and public health support since Jonah Wilson opened his original surgery?
- What other local medical provision has there been over the years through home visits, chemists, surgeries, hospitals, and in the gaol and the workhouse?
- What major medical and public health advances have taken place over the course of the period and what has been their impact locally?

Transactions of a Huntingdonshire Medical Society

The research about each successive generation of medical practitioners from 1821 to the present day has been made possible by the discovery of a manuscript in Huntingdon Library archives. This book, called *'Transactions'*, is a rare surviving transcript of the meetings of the Huntingdonshire Medical Society between 1793 and 1803. For many poorly qualified rural surgeons and apothecaries, such as those near Huntingdon and Godmanchester, the Medical Societies at the beginning of the 19th century represented a way of sharing notes and experiences of patient treatments that proved successful, or otherwise.

Although Jonah Wilson was never a member of the Medical Society, *Transactions* was passed to successive local medical practitioners following him in the 19th and 20th centuries. Each recipient was recognised by their peers as the most senior and expert as the emerging medical profession became established in the community.

Transactions provided the research outline for this project, along with the framed certificates of doctors' qualifications from the 19th century displayed at the Roman Gate surgery, along with other items from the Charles Hicks archives at the Practice in Huntingdon. Together, these enable us to identify past medical practitioners and the dates they were working in Huntingdon and Godmanchester as the Hicks Group Practice was established.

Each practitioner now forms the basis of a chapter of our book as 'men of their time' dealing with injuries, ailments and sickness in the local population. They used medical equipment and surgical techniques as they were being developed. They worked with local institutions providing medical and public health support up to and including, the foundation of the NHS. A final chapter brings us up to the present day. With the dates of their medical practice shown, they are:

- Jonah Wilson (1809 - 1848)
- Dr Michael Foster (1833 - 1876)
- Dr Herbert Lucas (1863 - 1919)
- Dr Charles Hicks (1910 - 1948)
- Dr Nelson Hicks (1947 - 1973)
- Dr Jim Rushton (1965 - 1995)

It was Dr Rushton of the Charles Hicks Practice who kindly donated *Transactions* to Huntingdon archives in April 2000, where it was later supplemented with a commentary by Arthur Rook.[1]

Chapter 1

Early medical practitioners in Huntingdonshire
Late 18th and early 19th century

In 1800, the combined population of Huntingdon and Godmanchester was under 4,000 (2,368 in Huntingdon and 1,573 in Godmanchester).[1] Huntingdonshire had an economy mostly based on agriculture with a rural population. The town of Huntingdon itself, was relatively prosperous with landowning gentry and the wealthier tradespeople owning 'many elegant houses.'[2] In Godmanchester there were some 'yeoman farmhouses'[3] but these were distinct from the homes of the largely agricultural labouring class, which in Godmanchester, as in parts of Huntingdon, was mostly the very poor,[4] and living in *'small, overcrowded cottages.'*[5]

Poverty and social class

Access to health care was largely dependent on ability to pay for treatment from a medical practitioner. Due to lack of medical knowledge at the time, this could produce *'uncertain results, and frequently cause discomfort or distress to the patient.'*[6] Another option for the gentry and more educated classes was to undertake *'a regimen of exercise, moderate diet and a judicious blend of business and pleasure.'*[7] In the 18th century this could involve 'taking the waters' in a spa town or a seaside resort, but again the results were variable, or some would say, imaginary.

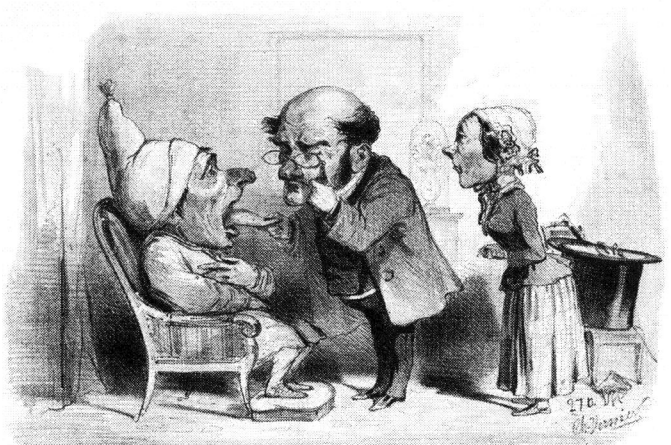

A physician examining a patient (Wellcome Collection)

For most people in all social classes, *'sickness remained a mysterious, often unpredictable and mostly unavoidable event, the result of blind fate or divine punishment.'*[8] Few were aware that disease could be spread by germs which thrived on dirt. Hand washing and bathing were largely unknown, so infectious diseases were common. These diseases would typically be classified as 'fever' (probably either typhus or typhoid) but also smallpox, measles, chicken pox or scarlet fever (all often confused with each other) or 'ague'.[9] Ague (malaria) was widely believed to be caused by 'bad air' or 'miasma', such as the *'pestiferous vapours and fogs'* identified in Wisbech.[10]

Apart from self-medication with herbal remedies or opiates, the poorest turned to the Poor Laws or medical charities for treatment. Those who could afford to, also used the services of a local medical practitioner with varying levels of quality, skills and accessibility.[11]

Medical practitioners

In eighteenth-century England, three main categories of medical practitioner existed, although in the provinces such as Huntingdonshire these distinctions were not always so clear. These categories are physicians, surgeons (or barber-surgeons) and apothecaries.

Physicians commanded most prestige as they were usually university educated. They largely followed classical theories of medicine based on 'humourism', which taught that the body contained four fluids, called humours – blood, yellow bile, black bile and phlegm. To be healthy, these needed to be kept in balance and this could be assessed by external physical symptoms.[12] They therefore checked the pulse of their wealthy patients and listened to their breathing, also checking skin, tongue and eyes for any discolouration, and then proceeded to prescribe. Early physicians often made a choice between 'conservative' options such as waiting and watching, herbal tonics, visit to a spa resort or simply bed rest. Alternatively, more 'heroic therapeutics' were used with patients who demanded (and could afford) results from bloodletting with leeches, violent purges and narcotics such as laudanum in order to restore 'balance'. Few, if any, of these therapies were clinically effective, and

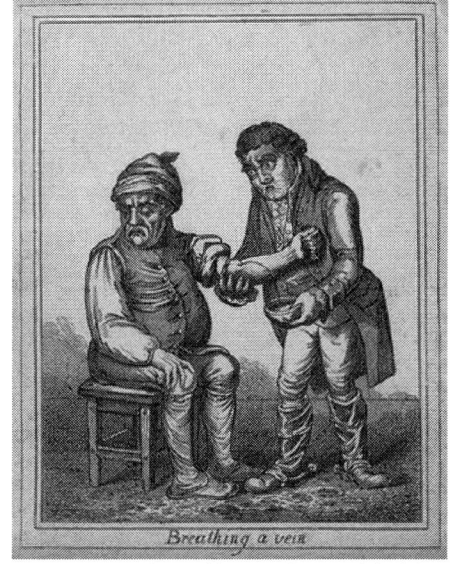

Drawing of an ill man being bled by a surgeon
(Wellcome Collection)

the essentials for commercial success as a physician have been described as *'a good reputation and a good horse'*.[13]

Surgeons were lower in the hierarchy and their activities were usually restricted to those that the physician did not perform – bloodletting, setting fractured limbs, lancing boils and pulling teeth for example. Only a few were skilled enough to perform amputations (without anaesthetic), or often crude forms of internal operation.[14] The traditional surgeon was often caricatured in periodicals and magazines as *'a man of the flesh – bold and beefy, handy with a knife and saw, little better than butchers and no more learned than barbers, with whose trade he frequently doubled.'*[15]

Apothecaries were originally seen primarily as tradesmen who mixed and dispensed the prescriptions of physicians. By the turn of the 19th century, they increasingly advised patients and prescribed medication. They often supplemented their income by operating from a retail shop, which in addition to ingredients for medicines, often sold tobacco as well as the cordials, herbs and elixirs used for self-medication such as Dr James's Powder for fever or Godfrey's Cordial for teething children.[16]

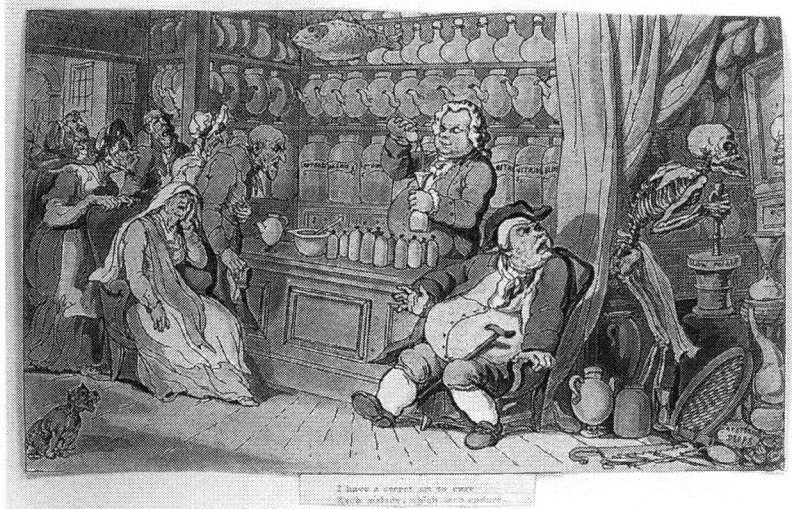

The dance of death: the apothecary (Wellcome Collection)

As well as the poor, women were largely excluded from care by medical practitioners, although rituals of childbirth were a shared heritage of women, regardless of social origin.[17] Childbirth included the presence of gossips, swaddling, and support for 'lying in'. This began to change in the 19th century with the increasing use of forceps as educated women demanded a better experience of childbirth, often with a physician or surgeon as 'man-midwife.'[18]

The Huntingdonshire Medical Society

It is difficult to estimate numbers of medical practitioners in Huntingdon in 1800, and from early records we only know of a few. Arthur Rook, in his book *Transactions of the Huntingdonshire Medical Society 1793-1803*, estimated that *'the area covered by an individual practitioner on horseback could rarely extend beyond 7 miles.'*[19] Little is known of Huntingdonshire Medical Society apart the transcript of the manuscript book *'Transactions'* (see Introduction) listing members of the Society and the minutes of their meetings.

None of the members of the Medical Society listed over the period lived in Huntingdon or Godmanchester. They were mostly surgeon-apothecaries, led by a physician, Dr Samuel Allvey of St Neots, meeting in each other's homes every 6 months. Other local practitioners that we do know, Mr Desborough in Huntingdon and Robert Fox in Godmanchester, appear not to have been members of the Society, or at least not at this date.

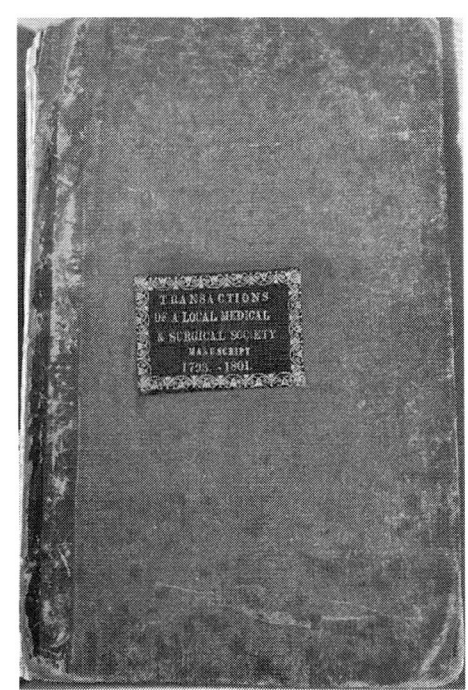

Front cover of 'Transactions of the Huntingdonshire Medical Society 1793 -1803'
(Courtesy Cambridgeshire Archives)

Cases outlied in 'Transactions' may have been representative of the members' experiences, although it may also be that personal interest or even 'shock value' had some part to play. Cases included cancer of the uterus, fungus of the elbow joint, scrophulous disease of the knee, a fractured cranium and tetanus.[20] Also recorded were a case of syphilis, treatment of typhus, a cataract operation, and a retained placenta.[21] Rather different to most cases presented to a GP in the Charles Hicks Practice in a typical day today!

The Dispensary

Members of the Huntingdonshire Medical Society would have charged for their services, sometimes just to cover the cost of medication but also for home visits and for their time.[22] However, for the poor of Huntingdon, there was another alternative source of help when the Dispensary opposite Mill Common was founded in 1789. This was one of the 38 general dispensaries established across England by 1800.[23] The Dispensary was essentially a charitable 'outpatient clinic' for those in the poor population able to attend in person. By the 1820s it was treating nearly 400 patients a year.[24] Funded through donations from the Earl of Sandwich, Lord Viscount Milton and James Rust (the Treasurer), the Dispensary was supported by annual subscriptions from the wealthy in the district.[25] (See Chapter 2)

Addenbrooke's Hospital

Addenbrooke's hospital was founded in 1766, following a charitable donation by John Addenbrooke. This was one of the first provincial hospitals founded following the model of five London hospitals opened between 1720 and 1745. Eleven patients were treated at Addenbrooke's in the first week but any records of these, and those patients that followed, will only reflect those who met the admission criteria at the time, and were able to pay, or classified as 'deserving poor' who could produce a letter signed by a wealthy sponsor.[26] In 1799-1800, seven Huntingdon parishes subscribed to use Addenbrooke's services, which may have included some out-patient services for those able to travel to Cambridge.[27]

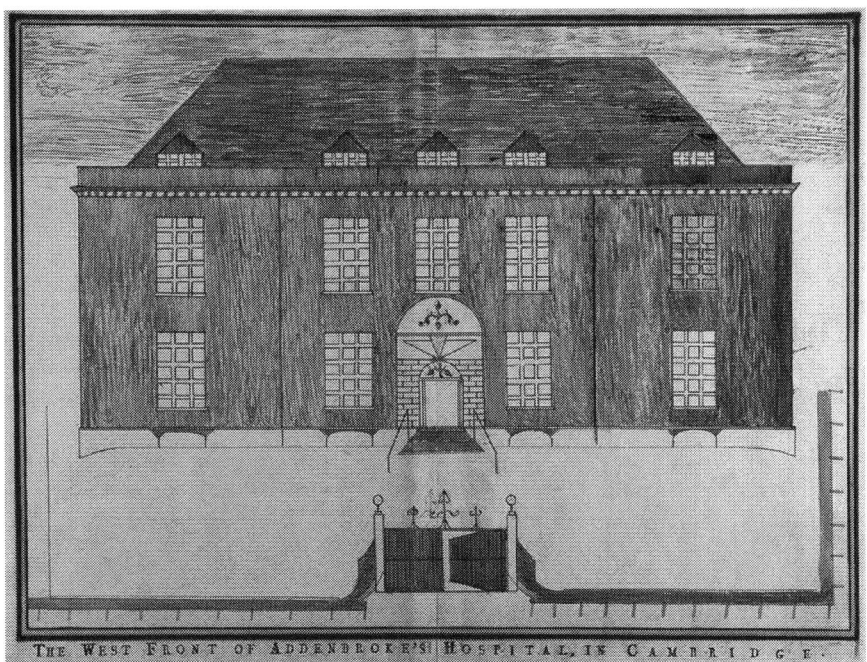

Drawing of the west front of Addenbrookes Hospital
(now the Judge Business School in Trumpington Street, Cambridge)
(Wellcome Collection)

Altruism and early professionalisation

The establishment of the first hospitals and dispensaries was intended to benefit the poorer population but for the rising medical profession it was 'a truly momentous event'.[28] Physicians and surgeons realized opportunities to observe and treat large numbers of patients and to dramatically increase understanding of disease. Ward journals and ledgers documented the success or failure of treatments, and medical journals and reference books began to be published. Voluntary hospitals such as Addenbrooke's enabled 'free' treatment of in-patients willing to become 'clinical objects.' The Anatomy Act of 1832 which allowed unclaimed bodies of deceased hospital patients to be used for demonstration or dissection in medical schools for surgical training is just one illustration of this process.[29]

Charlatans and quacks

Despite the growth of medical institutions enabling more effective treatment and sharing of medical knowledge, by 1809 it was estimated that charlatans and quacks outnumbered orthodox medical practitioners by a ratio of nine to one.[30] The medical journal, *The Lancet* founded in 1823, was concerned about '.....*the infatuated ignorance which prompts men to prefer the charlatan to the educated practitioner.*'[31] However, for most of the population, the nostrums and potions sold by quacks were a cheap means to self-help encouraged by handbills and newspaper advertisements promising quick cures to common afflictions such *as 'a fixed gout, dim eyes, asthma, the bile, the piles, and pain in the bowels and scurvy, and the smallpox prevented.*'[32]

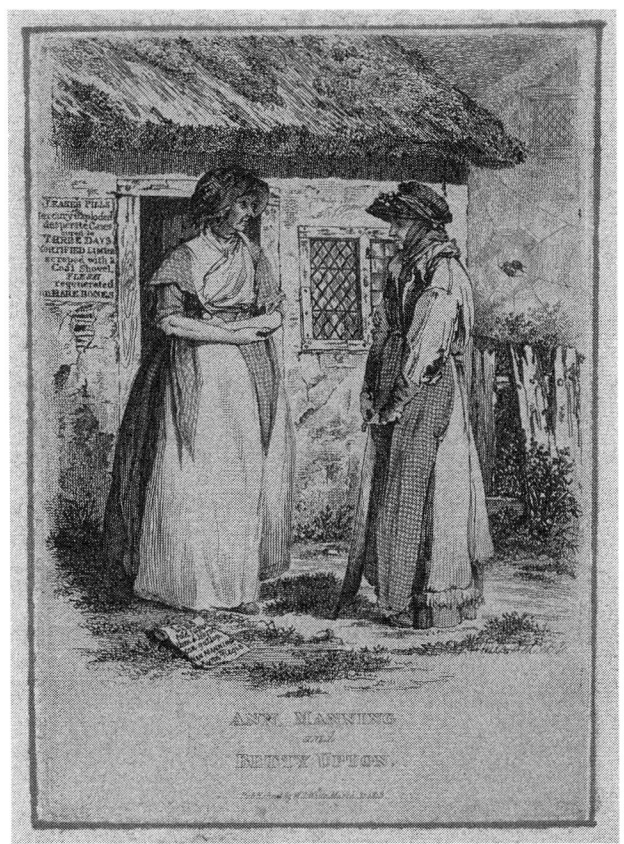

Anne Manning, a quack doctor, outside her cottage in 1818
(Wellcome Collection)

The notice on the wall next to Anne Manning reads:
- Leakes Pills.
- Desperate cases cured in three days.
- Mortified limbs scraped with a coal shovel.
- Flesh regenerated on bare bones.

In the next Chapter we look at how the more professional practice of medicine in Huntingdon began to develop.

Chapter 2

Jonah Wilson (1809–1848)
Early medical practice in Huntingdon

Jonah Wilson is named at the centre of the plaque in the painting at Roman Gate surgery in Godmanchester. His medical practice was established in Huntingdon town square in 1821. In early 19th century provincial towns, distinctions between apothecary and surgeon were less rigidly applied and there was no clear distinction between those qualified or unqualified.[1] Jonah Wilson never gained formal qualifications but established a well-regarded medical practice in Huntingdon.

In 1820 the combined population of Huntingdon and Godmanchester was 5,130 – an increase of over 20% since 1800. Demand for medical treatment was growing from the newly educated middle class as well as an emerging awareness among business owners of the benefits of enabling workers to stay healthy and productive.[2] As the medical market expanded, new practitioners such as Wilson arrived in rural towns and sought new patients with an increased range of medical services on offer.[3]

There is evidence of other barber-surgeons already working in Huntingdon in the 18th century, including William Smith, who was given the body of a murderer called Richard Keen to *'be dissected and anatomised'*.[4] Using bodies of murderers for study was customary before the Anatomy Act of 1832. Another Huntingdon surgeon, Mr Desborough, was prison surgeon at the County Gaol (or Bridewell) at the turn of the century.[5]

Early training

Born in 1778 in Oswaldkirk in Yorkshire, Wilson had been apprenticed to his uncle Mr Wass of Thirsk, *'a very respectable practitioner of medicine'*.[6] Wilson studied briefly in Edinburgh and began working as an apothecary in St Neots in the 1790s. He recognised that to establish himself as a competitive medical practitioner, he needed to broaden his knowledge and skills in surgery.

Wilson moved to 'hospital practice' at Guy's Hospital, working under Sir Astley Cooper. Cooper had attended lectures in Paris where the medical school recognised the significance of practical training in surgery.

Astley Cooper was *'the most famous surgeon of his generation'*[7], becoming surgeon to George IV and Queen Victoria. Cooper emphasised to students such as Wilson, not only the value of first-hand experience of surgery through observation at post-mortems but also a wider understanding of medicine and pharmacy.[8] He commented, *'the study of medicine is important to the surgeon; he should be able to prescribe with certainty.'*[9]

Establishing a Huntingdon practice

Returning to Huntingdon to join Mr Desborough, Wilson became prison surgeon in 1809 and expanded the Practice, moving to the Market Square in 1821. Wilson had not qualified following the Apothecaries Act of 1815,[10] but well understood anatomy and surgery from his time with Sir Astley Cooper. Like many surgeon-apothecaries at the time, he would have visited sick and dying patients in their homes and responded to emergencies such as wounds and fractured bones, performing amputations without anaesthetic when necessary.[11] Working in a rural area like Huntingdon where medical and surgical knowledge was poorly understood, Wilson was much sought after and trebled the financial returns from Mr Desborough's practice in the first year.

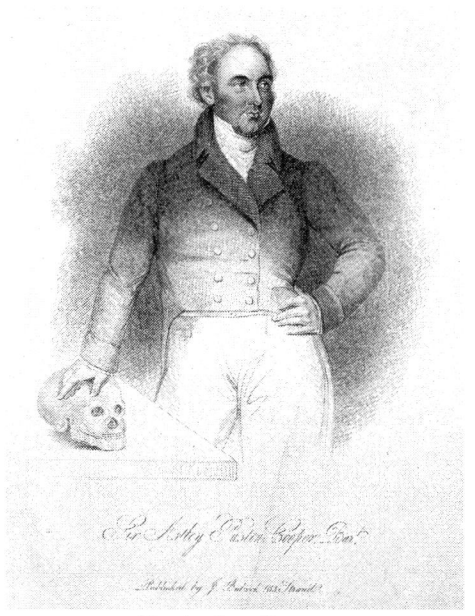

Sir Astley Cooper
(Wellcome Collection)

He also continued as an apothecary and was renowned for his knowledge of pharmacy, publishing *'Pharmacopoeia Chirurgica'* in 1809.[12] His prescriptions were considered *'models worthy of notice and imitation'* and, as he had the necessary knowledge and skills to formulate and manufacture the required tablets, within a few years the practice was the most lucrative in the neighbourhood.[13] Wilson worked the practice single-handedly for 12 years until joined by newly qualified Michael Foster as his assistant in 1833.

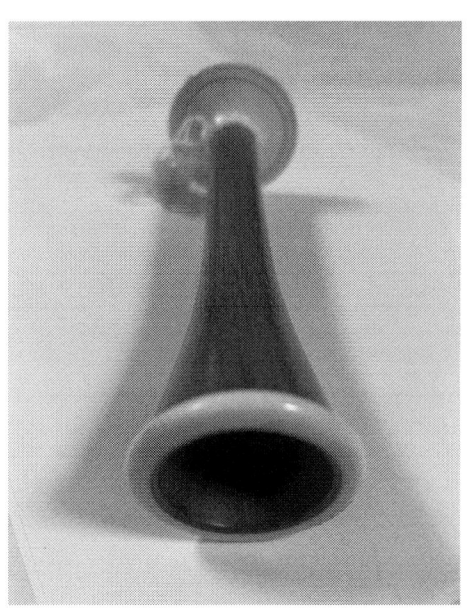

An early wooden stethoscope
(Courtesy of Thackray Museum of Medicine)

Wilson would have been among the first medical practitioners in Huntingdon to use a stethoscope. Invented in France in 1816 by Rene Laennec, it was a wooden instrument for listening to a patient's chest, particularly those suffering from tuberculosis (TB). Treatment for TB at the time, often involved a 'low diet and bloodletting'.[14] Use of leeches for bloodletting was a common treatment used by apothecaries and was considered beneficial for most medical conditions.

The Huntingdon Dispensary

By 1820 access to Huntingdon Dispensary was limited due to rising demand for treatment. Patients were admitted every Saturday at Mr Bates' shop, the druggist, and those unable to attend were visited in their homes by the physician.[15] In 1823, the physician was Dr Morton, supported by Surgeons Wilson, Oakley and Leslie.[16]

Records from Peterborough Dispensary show treatments at the time ranged from standard bloodletting with leeches, to trusses for hernias, medications for fevers and prescribing of epsom salts, laudanum, quinine and opium powder.[17] Huntingdon records indicate there was a minor surgery, including amputations and even use of an unidentified 'electrical machine'.[18]

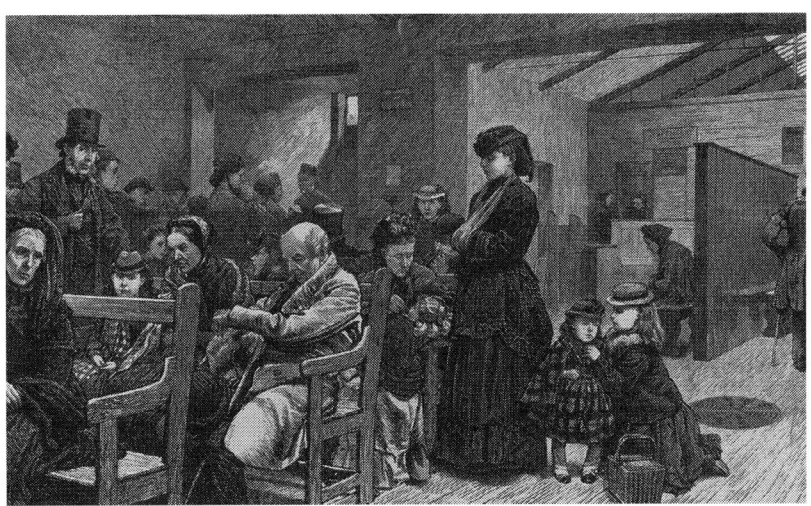

Dispensary waiting room
(Wellcome Collection)

Medical staff other than the physicians were unpaid, but their presence added status to the Dispensary, attracting new benefactors. Also, the physicians and surgeons *'were sensitized to the problems of the lower classes, especially the relationship between unhealthy environments and contagious fevers.'*[19] Through the Dispensary the working-class became more aware of personal hygiene and women in households could gain some support and possibly respite, for their home-based care of family members and neighbours.[20]

In 1831 an 'infirmary house' (later known as All Saints Rectory on the Walks) was added to Huntingdon Dispensary on Mill Common. Records show that in 1833, 64 patients received treatment in the infirmary, 36 were cured, 3 relieved, 1 discharged, 8 were 'incurable', 2 died and 6 were still inmates.[21] Patients were not allowed to drink alcohol, smoke, swear or leave the premises. Those occupying the few available beds long term were charged one shilling per week for food and laundry.[22] Additional staff by 1831, included the physician Dr John Baumgartner from Godmanchester and William Ward, newly arrived in Huntingdon.[23]

Smallpox vaccinations

By 1831 one common treatment at the Huntingdon Dispensary, was smallpox vaccinations. Since the seventeenth century, smallpox had been the most feared, widespread and fatal infection in England. The disease was passed between people by droplet infection – sneezing and coughing. There had been outbreaks of infection in Cambridgeshire throughout the 18th century. Infection quickly spread with increasing travel as road networks improved.

Inoculation began in England in the 1720s by deliberately infecting a healthy person with smallpox 'pus' from someone suffering a mild form of the disease. This appeared to give immunity but was not always successful and was usually restricted to wealthier clients. Many were influenced by Lady Mary Montague (of Hinchingbrooke House), who had observed this technique in Turkey, while her husband was the British Ambassador in Constantinople in 1716.[24]

In 1798 Edward Jenner advocated an alternative approach using 'vaccination' with cowpox to prevent smallpox infection as a simpler, quicker and cheaper alternative. By 1801 over 100,000 people had been vaccinated. In 1807 Parliament required the Royal College of Physicians to organise vaccinations across the country and by 1819 Robert Fox was administering smallpox vaccinations in Godmanchester.

Vaccination was not always locally accepted. Nelson Hicks argued in his lecture on the History of Medicine that:

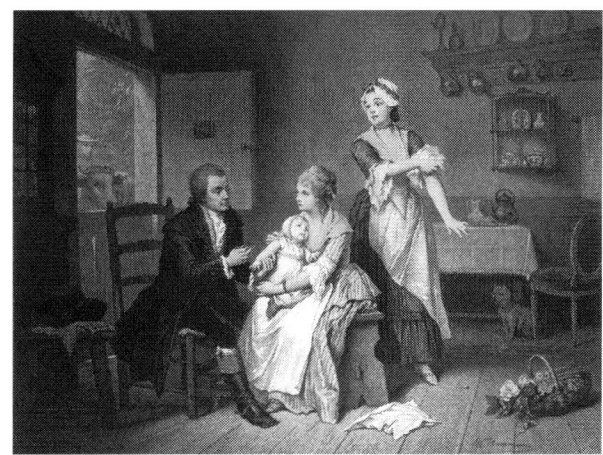

Edward Jenner vaccinating his infant son
(Wellcome Collection)

"Smallpox was only slowly coming under control as vaccination was superseding the more 'heroic' inoculation technique still practiced in the 1830s and 1840s in Huntingdon,

it being still considered that you were not immune until you had been exposed to infection. Many children were taken to a sick friend's house and had the smallpox exudate (pus) rubbed on their arms to make sure they were properly immune."[25]

The Dispensary continued adult vaccination until 1853 when the Town and County Hospital was founded. In 1840 inoculations were declared illegal and in 1852 vaccinations became compulsory in Britain. This programme was strictly enforced until 1887 with subsequent Huntingdon doctors including Herbert Lucas (Chapter 4) taking on the role of 'Public Vaccinator'. This led to a drop in deaths from smallpox and no epidemic has been reported in England since 1934.[26]

The County Prison (Gaol)

Wilson was surgeon to the County Gaol in Huntingdon for over 30 years until joined by Michael Foster in 1841. His attendance was three times a week, and more often if required. His salary was £20 per year plus half a guinea additional for itch and venereal cases, and 5 shillings for attending corporal punishment cases.

'Very often the surgeon had to contend with 'low diseases' which he put down to the humidity of the prison. One of these was ague (malaria). His main struggle, however, was to keep men who had been sentenced to hard labour, healthy on a minimal diet. He operated a kind of seesaw of extra diet and remission of labour to achieve this.'[27]

Wilson also occasionally treated scurvy in men who had been in prison for over six months. It was possible to be close to death with scurvy, and he once saved a man's life from the disease with a treatment of port and lemon. Small beer would have been a good addition to the diet as a preventative measure in his opinion, and after six months in the prison he had to order it as extra diet in six out of ten cases.[28]

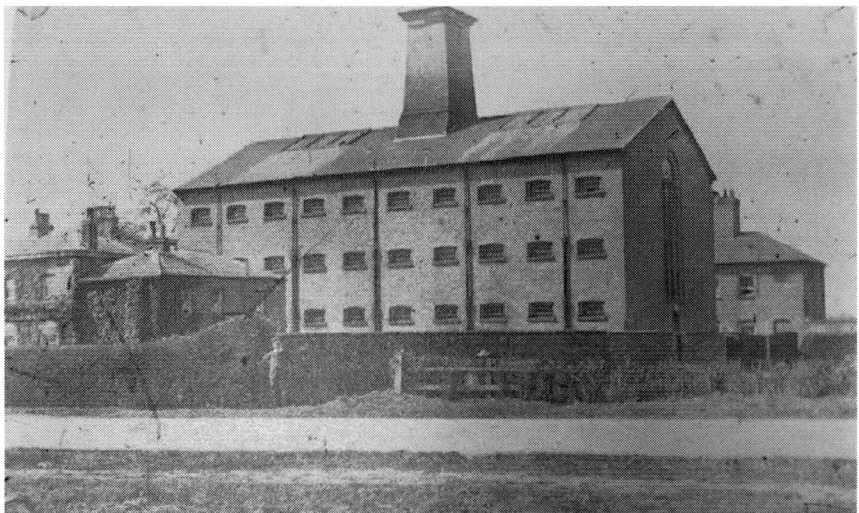

Huntingdon County Gaol and Bridewell, St Peter's Road (1828 -1886)
(Courtesy Cambridgeshire Archives)

Obituary

Wilson never became a member of the Royal College of Surgeons. He also rejected the offer of a degree of Doctor of Medicine (MD) from Aberdeen. He was distraught at the premature death of his son, who intended to follow him in medicine and suffering from depression and gout he left Huntingdon 1848 and died in 1851, aged 73. Jonah Wilson's obituary notice in the *Provincial Medical and Surgical Journal* noted that he was,

> *'ready to perform an operation when necessary, yet fondly admired for reliance upon nature's great powers. He was remarkably successful in surgical cases; his knowledge of midwifery, in all its mechanical forms and vital powers, was complete. Few men of his day were his equal.'*[29]

There are no records of Wilson joining Huntingdonshire Medical Society. This is probably why William Ward received the Society minutes of 'Transactions' instead. Subsequently, this was passed to Michael Foster who is the subject of Chapter 3.

Other local medical practitioners

Robert Fox

Robert Fox was parish surgeon of Godmanchester. Fox trained in medicine and became a member of the Royal College of Surgeons (MRCS) in 1819. He practised in both Huntingdon and Godmanchester and was prominent in Huntingdonshire Medico-Chirurgical Society (the likely successor organisation to the Huntingdonshire Medical Society). He administered the first smallpox vaccinations in Godmanchester in 1819 and was a member of the 'Cholera committee' in 1832. He was a bailiff of the Borough in 1831–32 and Medical Officer of Health to administer the Poor Law Amendment Act from 1834. Robert Fox died in 1843 aged 45, *'greatly esteemed for his benevolence'*. [30]

William Ward

William Ward was given the manuscript of 'Transactions' in 1864 by Thomas Smith of Peterborough. Ward was a member of the 'opposing partnership' to Jonah Wilson.[31] He qualified as an apothecary (LSA) and surgeon (MRCS) in 1823 from Guy's and St. Thomas's Hospitals in London. His Practice was in Huntingdon. He was a surgeon to the Infirmary and Dispensary and later became one of the first Medical Officers to the County Hospital. He was elected President of the Literary and Scientific Institution in Huntingdon and hosted its opening in the Commemoration Hall in 1842 with a eulogy from Robert Fox.[32] He died in retirement in 1873.

Chapter 3

Dr Michael Foster (1833–1876)
Cholera and early general practice

The population of Huntingdon increased to over 3,500 in the 1830s (Godmanchester was by now 2,100) and more medical practitioners began to establish themselves in the town. Michael Foster is the next link in the chain of those who inherited 'The Transactions of the Huntingdonshire Medical Society'. He is a key figure in the development of general medical practice and healthcare in Huntingdon and Godmanchester.

Early years

Foster was born in 1810, at Holywell, near Hitchin. His father was a yeoman farmer from a puritan background. In 1826, aged 16, he was apprenticed to Mr Peck, a surgeon from Kimbolton. An apprenticeship was *the 'time-honoured route to the apothecary's trade or the surgeon's craft, reflecting an established system for passing on the skills of one generation of experts to another.'*[1] By living in his master's house, the apprentice gained a thorough understanding of a practical medical life. This was important as Foster was from a non-medical family. Foster learned well from Mr Peck and in 1831, he entered University College Hospital, London, where in 1833, he qualified as a surgeon (MRCS) and gained his licence as an apothecary (LSA).

In 1833 Foster joined Jonah Wilson in Huntingdon, firstly as assistant and then as partner. He married Mercy Cooper and had a family of ten children: his eldest son, Michael Foster Jnr. (1836-1907), became a famous physiologist. By 1841, census records show Michael Foster and his family living in Brampton Road with three servants and an apprentice, John Lloyd.

Cholera epidemic of 1832

'In 1841, household density in Godmanchester averaged 4.56 persons. The small cottages were acutely overcrowded and in one case 2 adults and 8 children, slept in one small room.'[2] The consequence for the spread of disease in such conditions was soon to become apparent.

A cholera epidemic had arrived in Huntingdon by 1832. As a new disease in England, physicians were unfamiliar with its causes or treatment. Contemporary medical opinion was that cholera was caused by bad air or 'miasma' from dung heaps, sewers, damp and dirt. Others argued it was caused from contact with diseased people through overcrowding. A 'Pest House' had already been built in Huntingdon on Spring Common in the 1760s to isolate smallpox sufferers. In the 1830s it was also used to house a few cholera patients whose homes were considered inadequate.[3]

Cholera spread rapidly amongst the poor, who were often instructed to avoid alcohol and eat moderately. Patients were often bled with leeches or were medicated with camphor and mercury with little effect. These treatments just weakened the bodies of those suffering from cholera and caused them to become even more dehydrated, hastening death within 2 to 6 days from infection in many cases.[4]

In 1832 there were over 56,000 deaths from suspected cholera in the United Kingdom. Cholera was widespread in Huntingdonshire with its many poor inhabitants and low-lying ponds, lakes and bad drainage. Nelson Hicks recorded in his lecture:

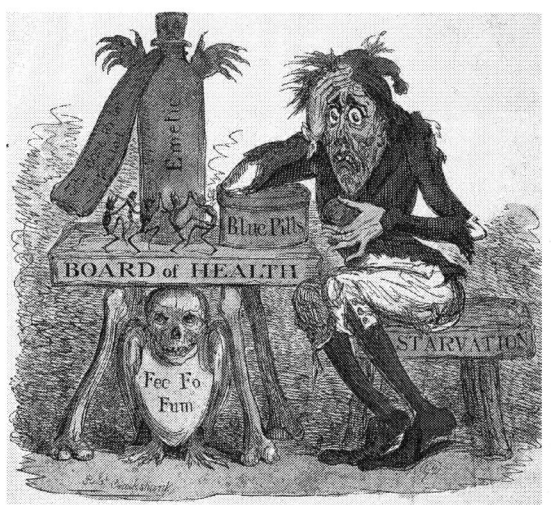
A cholera patient experimenting with 'remedies' (Wellcome Collection)

> *"In Fenstanton out of 1000 population, 100 died. In Ramsey where it was very bad, all business and markets closed, and in the town, parents forsook their children and young adults their parents as soon as they were attacked."*[5]

Attempting to control the disease, the government established local Boards of Health. Despite their efforts, there were further outbreaks of cholera in East Anglia in 1848, 1849, 1853 and 1854. In Germany, Johann Peter Frank had established a comprehensive overview of the links between public health and hygiene as early as 1779.[6] However in the UK, it was Dr John Snow's work in London in 1849, that provided proof that cholera was a water-borne infection that could be controlled by a pure water supply and good sewerage systems.[7] A report by Edwin Chadwick on 'The Sanitary Conditions of the Labouring Population of Great Britain' in 1842 further highlighted the links between poor living conditions, disease, and high mortality rates. This report informed the First Public Health Act in 1848 with which Michael Foster became involved.

The workhouse and the prison

The 1834 Poor Law Amendment Act had abolished the old system of 'outdoor relief' and formalised a system of workhouses. Godmanchester and Huntingdon became part of the Huntingdon Union, and a new workhouse was built in 1837 on the corner of St Peter's Road and Ermine Street in Huntingdon. By 1862 there were 228 inmates.[8] Foster would have been one of the surgeons attending to the health of both male and female workhouse occupants.

From 1841 to 1844, Foster was also surgeon to Huntingdon County prison, along with Jonah Wilson. He then took over the role for the next 22 years, sharing it with Herbert Lucas from 1866 until 1876, when it was taken over completely by Herbert Lucas (see Chapter 4). Foster may not have regarded this role as a top priority since, *'In 1842 the Inspector recorded that the surgeon visited the prison daily but did not comply with the Gaol Acts by seeing each prisoner twice a week and did not necessarily visit those in solitude.'*[9]

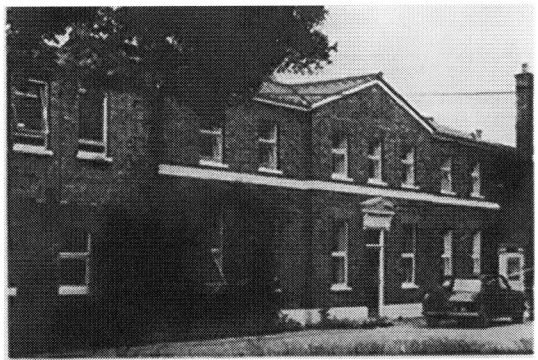

Huntingdon Union workhouse – later converted to Walnut Tree House and after 1948, Petersfield Hospital.
(Courtesy Cambridge Community Archive Network)

The First Public Health Act of 1848

Despite declining cholera infections, medical challenges continued because of poor water supplies. The Public Health Act encouraged (but did not enforce) local authorities to provide water at public expense. In Godmanchester, Michael Green noted:

> 'The absence of any drainage, apart from two ancient ditches, the town drain and the parish drain and the lack of 'privvies', made the town in flood-time one large open cesspool. The shallow wells which supplied all the drinking water were contaminated and in 1847-8 one-ninth of Godmanchester's population was suffering from typhoid or similar infection.'[10]

Foster gave evidence to William Lee's report to the General Board of Health. This enquiry into the sewerage, water supply and sanitary condition in Godmanchester proved to be a turning point in local public health. He recorded his experience of diseases in Godmanchester:

> *"From my experience during the last five years, fever is constantly present and, of course, increasing in extent and virulence during epidemics. I have attended more cases of fever in Godmanchester than in all other places put together within my practice, except the Union workhouse."*[11]

William Lee's final report made recommendations for better water supply, improved town drainage, embankment of the river Ouse, improved pavements and 'public cleansing' (waste collection). However, several improvements took 80 years to be implemented. Initially a Local Board of Health was established, and in 1853 a main drainage system was provided. However, piped water was not supplied in Godmanchester until 1936.[12]

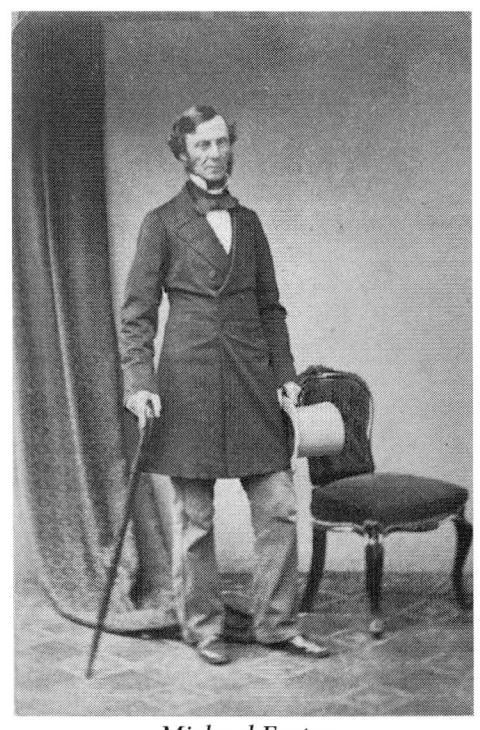

Michael Foster
(Courtesy of Cambridgeshire Archives)

An established Huntingdon Practice

Foster took over the Practice when Jonah Wilson retired in 1848. Census records for 1851 show that he is listed as a surgeon/apothecary and his family was now living in his Practice premises in 35 Huntingdon High Street. He had 2 apprentices as surgeon/apothecaries, William Cooper (age 16) and George Coleman (age 18).

Some of Michael Foster's medical equipment is in the Norris Museum in St Ives. The contents of a typical medical chest from this period are a rather terrifying glimpse of treatment available – and the types of surgery being performed before the use of anaesthetic was widespread.

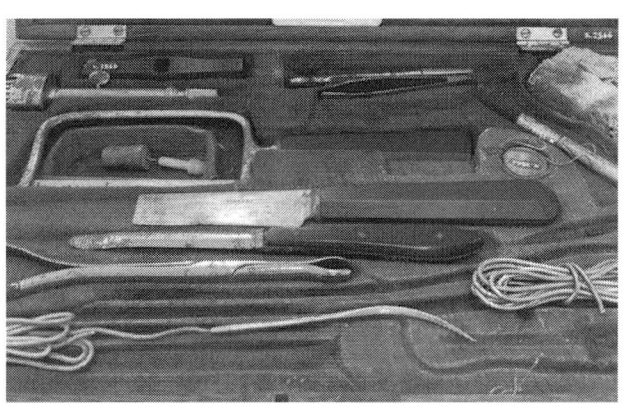

A 19th century surgery set
(Courtesy of the Norris Museum)

In 1846 Robert Liston began to use ether as a sedative during surgery and in 1847 James Simpson (one of Lister's students) discovered the preferable use of chloroform as an anaesthetic.[13]

Michael Foster owned a 'tracheotomy set in a mahogany case' and an 'ophthalmoscope with a candle stick and lens', both in the Norris Museum. Operations by surgeons to free breathing blockages and treat cataracts were quite common. It is not known however, when and to what extent, Foster adopted the use of anaesthetics.

The Medical Act of 1858

The 1858 Medical Act established the General Medical Council (GMC) which still exists today. The Act required doctors to be registered with the GMC to qualify for income from appointment as a Poor Law Medical Officer, or new posts such as a Medical Officer of Public Health or Certifying Factory Surgeon.

Michael Foster was elected to Fellowship of the Royal College of Surgeons (FRCS) in 1852. He was given 'Transactions' by William Ward at around this time establishing a clear link through the next 150 years to the Hicks Group Practice today.

A New Hospital for Huntingdon

In 1851 Dr Ward and Mr Foster presented to the Infirmary committee the 'painful inadequacy' of the Infirmary House as well as the *'great advantage that would result to the poorer classes if a larger building could be constructed for twenty beds.'*[14] This was to become the new County Hospital in 1853.

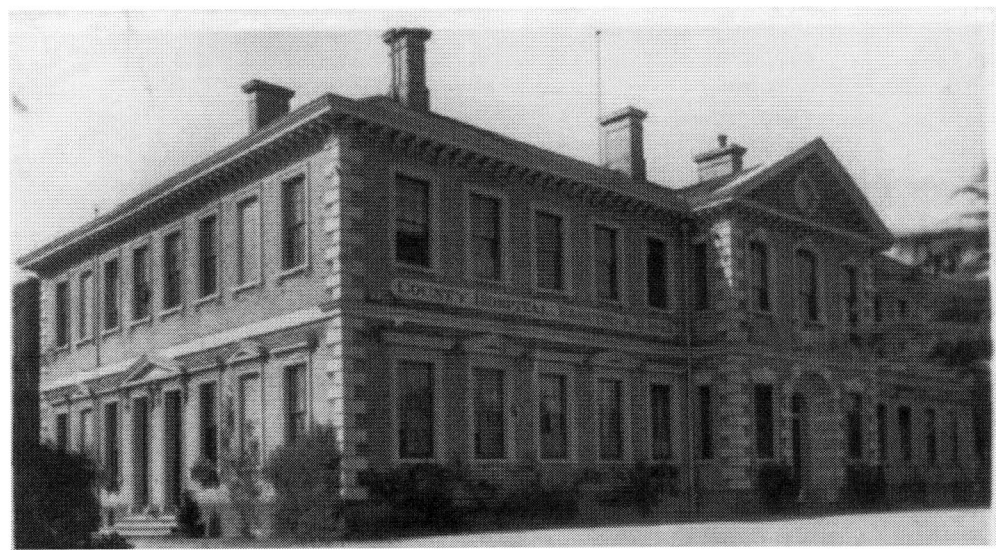

Huntingdon County Hospital (Courtesy Cambridge Community Archive Network)

It was agreed that if £4,000 could be raised by public subscription, then James Rust (the Treasurer) would contribute £1,000, so with cash in hand, the total would be £7,000. The new hospital was on the site of the Dispensary on Mill Common. There were 4 wards (2 male and 2 female) with 26 beds, a dispensary, a drug store, 2 consulting rooms, a surgeon's room, a sleeping room for the surgeon, an apartment for the matron, and a committee room, together with kitchens and offices.

Medical staff in the Hospital when it opened were:

- Dr Baumgartner (physician) who had trained in medicine at Edinburgh University and held clinics for the local poor in his mews at Island Hall in Godmanchester.
- William Ward MD and FRCS (physician and consulting surgeon).
- Michael Foster (surgeon).
- Wotton Isaacson (surgeon).[15]

Increasing competition

The Medical Act, a new Hospital and the development of specialist instruments such as medical thermometers and stethoscopes, all contributed to improved health care in the community.

The English physician Sir Thomas Allbutt developed the first practical medical thermometer as it became clear that extremes of temperature could help diagnose specific illnesses. Allbutt's thermometer was able to record a patient's temperature in 5 minutes and was widely used from the mid-19th century onwards.

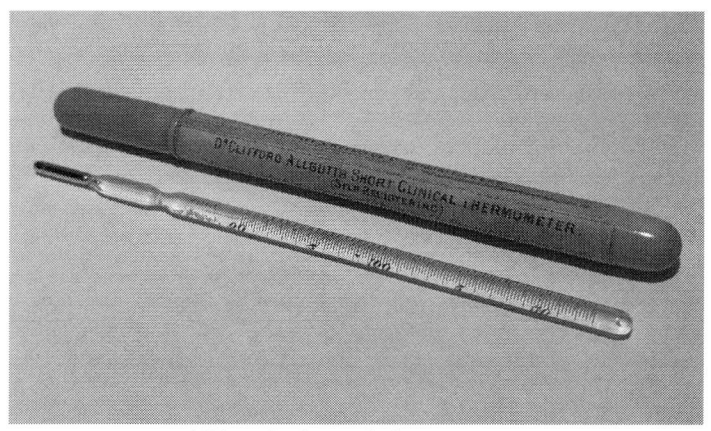

Allbutt's clinical thermometer
(Courtesy of Thackray Museum of Medicine)

Qualified medical practitioners such as Foster faced increasing competition. Not only unlicensed practitioners (despite the 1858 Medical Act), but druggists, chemists and the variety of 'quacks' continued to grow. In Huntingdon by 1854, several chemists had established themselves in the High Street. These included Isaac Bentham, William Bryant, William Ekins (chemist and soda water maker), George Lewis (chemist and druggist) and John Provost (chemist and soda water maker).[16] As well as soda water, these druggists supplied a range of medications such as the ever-popular Daffy's Elixir for digestive problems (sometimes 'diluted' with gin), Fenning's Children's Cooling Powders or Godfrey's Cordial for teething babies and children (a mixture of laudanum and sweet syrup).[17] These were sold alongside newer speciality products such as cod-liver oil, malt extract and blackcurrant throat sweets – known as 'pastilles' from the French for medicinal pill. [18]

Itinerant 'quacks' also came to Huntingdon on market days. Cures for common afflictions were promoted with handbills and newspaper advertisements.[19] Which specific medication, ointment or powder would be sold for each of these is now sometimes unclear, but the quack salesman would have the solution as *'all are easily cured, and the smallpox prevented.'*[20]

Poorer communities in rural Huntingdonshire villages continued with even cheaper local 'cures' such as keeping the foot of a mole in a pocket to cure rheumatism, wrapping a dirty sock round the neck to cure a sore throat,

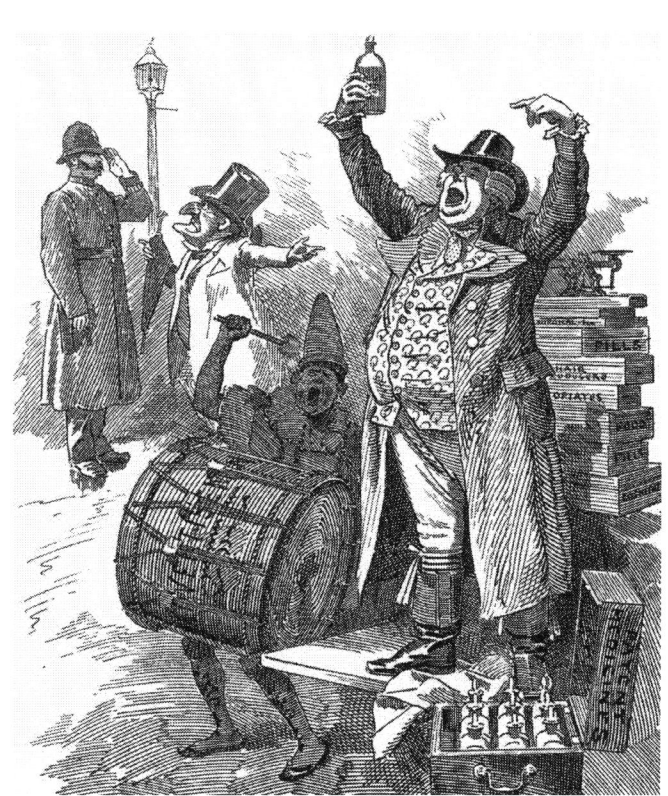

A Quack selling his potions
(Wellcome Collection)

keeping guinea pigs to ward off smallpox[21] or a Fenland special; to *'keep a wrap of dried tobacco round the wrist'* to avoid the ague.'[22] Scientific medicine was clearly not yet well established.

Professional development

In 1861 Michael Foster was elected President of the Cambridge and Huntingdon branch of the British Medical Association (BMA). Still living and working from 35 High Street, Huntingdon, he now had another 16 year-old apprentice, John Leigh. Foster is clearly successful by this time with established sources of income from his roles at the Hospital, Poor Law Union, the County Gaol and the workhouse.[23] As a Medical Officer for the Poor Law, after 1865 he was also entitled to keep 'one man servant, one horse, and a two or four wheeled carriage, free from assessed taxes.'[24]

He appears to have had good relationships with other influential local medical practitioners such as William Ward, Wotton Isaacson and William Morriston Davis. Herbert Lucas (Chapter 4) joined him as a partner in the practice in 1863. Such partnerships became increasingly common towards the middle of the century as patient demands and workloads increased.[26]

Foster became most prosperous from his private clients. He fits the description of doctors given by Nelson Hicks *as "on foot in the town with country visits on horseback or in a gig or dogcart."* He would have been increasingly sought after as *"he now had a means of alleviating pain. He had anaesthetics that he could use. He could obtain morphia, atropine and strychnine in reasonably stable forms, and the new hypodermic syringe had been invented in 1850. He could also obtain chloroform and ether which was usually administered on a pad of cotton wool in a tumbler, and with remarkable abandon as time went on."*[27]

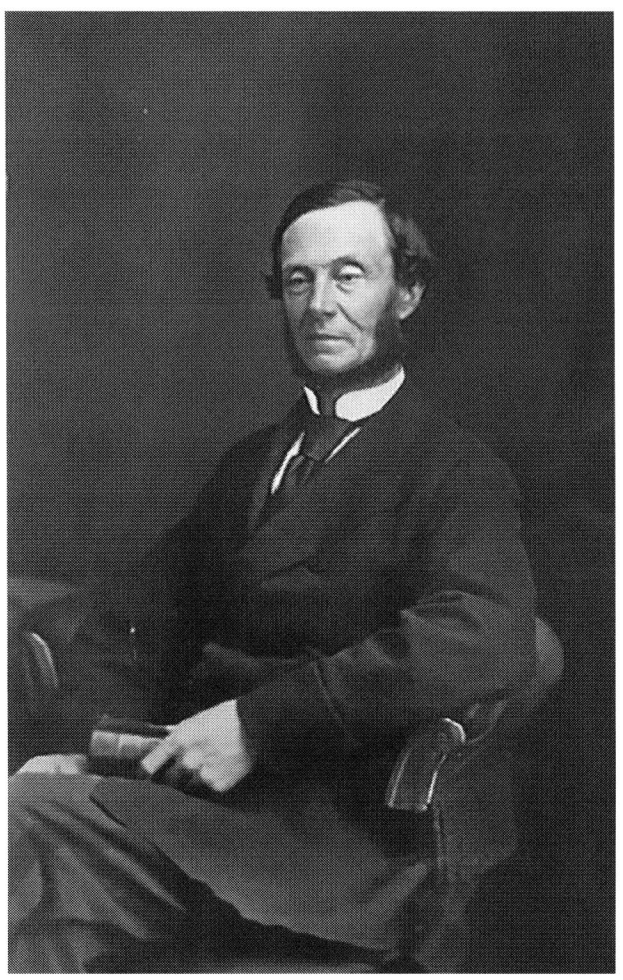

Michael Foster showing the importance of the 'identifiable garb' to display professional status.[25]
(Courtesy of the Norris Museum)

Alexander Wood, a Scottish physician, invented the first hypodermic needle that used a true syringe and hollow needle in 1853. His model was widely adopted in England.

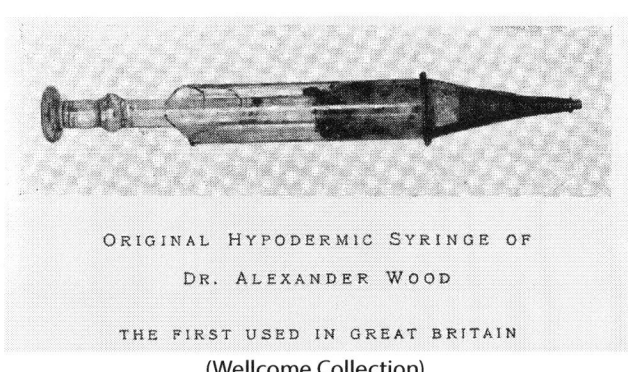

(Wellcome Collection)

Foster is described as *'winning from his patients not only an almost unbounded confidence in his professional skill, but also a strong personal affection, growing out of his blameless, unselfish character and pure Christian spirit'*.[28]

A new Medico-Chirurgical Society in Huntingdon

In 1847 Michael Foster had founded (and was President of) a Medico-Chirurgical Society in Huntingdon. Proceedings of the Society were researched by Dr Jesse Garrood of Alconbury (and later, the Huntingdonshire Cyclists Battalion), the son in law of the Society's original secretary. These records have been summarised by Arthur Rook.[29]

Foster's Presidential address on his retirement in 1876 emphasised the lack of important medical advances and although he himself was conscious of change, the change was rather in the approach to disease and to diagnosis rather than *'materia medica'* (i.e. the drugs used in their treatment'). Many treatments had by now been proven, such as use of quinine for ague, and later used by Dr Garrood to attempt to alleviate symptoms of 'Spanish Flu' in 1918. However, the real advances had been *"the extraordinary means for diagnosis such as stethoscopes for chest diseases, microscopes for urinary disease and ophthalmoscopes for eyes and thermometers for fevers."* Members of the Huntingdon Society appear to have been in advance of their contemporaries and many successors, in their attitude to less use of blood-letting and the relative simplicity of their prescriptions.[30]

Later life

Foster stayed true to his religious roots, being described as *'a well-liked and skilful surgeon'*, whilst known for being a *'strangely non-conformist radical on politics and religion.'*[31] In 1871 he was still living in the High Street along with Michael Foster Jnr. (age 35) now a well-established Professor of Physiology. Also in the house were other children and grandchildren, plus Arthur Wagstaffe, an apprentice and three domestic servants. He began to suffer 'transient pains' which were followed by the unmistakeable symptoms of 'paralysis agitans', or Parkinson's disease. Despite the best efforts of his family and professional friends, he died in 1880 and is buried in Priory cemetery in Huntingdon. Of his family of ten children, only three (Michael Foster Jnr. and two daughters) survived him, along with Mercy, his wife.[32]

A famous son

The son of Michael Foster Snr. was Sir Michael Foster KCB, FRS, VMH, the eminent physiologist. Born in 1836 in Huntingdon, educated at Huntingdon Grammar School, he studied medicine at the University of London and became the Member of Parliament for London University.

He was instrumental in organising the Cambridge Biological School, also Professor of Practical Physiology University College, London and Secretary of the Royal Society. He died in 1907 and is buried in Huntingdon cemetery.

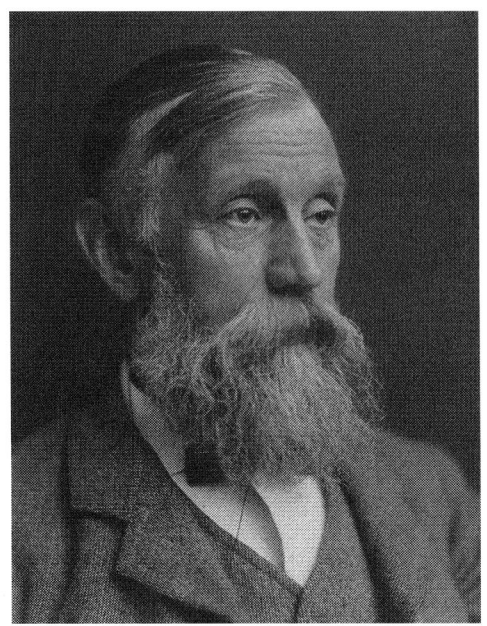

Sir Michael Foster
(Wellcome Collection)

Other local medical practitioners

William Ward (see Chapter 2)

Wotton Isaacson

Isaacson practiced in Huntingdon and by 1851 had a surgery in the High Street. He was a qualified surgeon (MRCS) and married William Ward's daughter, Elizabeth. Elizabeth was only 32 when Isaacson died in 1859 aged 45, leaving assets of less than £1500. Elizabeth continued to live with William Ward and his family, along with her 2 daughters.

Edmund Carver

Born 1824, he was a qualified surgeon and apothecary. He gained a BA in 1858 and Bachelor of Medicine (MB) in 1859. He became a Doctor of Medicine (MD) in 1891. After a period at Brompton Hospital for Consumption, he became House Surgeon at Addenbrooke's Hospital. Attracted by the offer of a partnership with William Ward in 1866, after Wotton Isaacson's death, he moved to Huntingdon and was appointed Surgeon to the County Hospital.

Chapter 4

Dr Herbert Lucas (1863–1919)
Establishing public health in Huntingdon

Herbert Lucas continued medical developments and oversaw public health improvements into the 20th century. He was born 1843 in Hitchin. Little is known about his family, early childhood or education. He came to Huntingdon and joined Michael Foster in his medical practice in 1863, probably as an apprentice or (more common by this date) to receive a practical education as a 'medical pupil' by working as an assistant. This was a common route into a country practice, especially for those not born into medical families. It was outlawed in 1892, after which time a professional qualification was required to legally practice medicine.[1]

It is estimated that in the 1860s at least 20% of practices employed assistants, often at a salary as low as £30 per year. Lucas's role in Dr Foster's practice can be seen by the requirements needed to apply for an assistant's place since *'typically, an ability to ride a horse (later bicycle) was seen to be near essential, and neat hand was useful for keeping the books.'*[2] Assistants were also required to mix and dispense medicines and sometimes visit and treat patients.

A General Practitioner in Huntingdon

Lucas progressed to training at Guy's Hospital in London and qualified as an apothecary (LSA) and surgeon (MRCS) in 1865. Lucas was now well equipped with the necessary medical skills for the challenges that awaited him as one of the next generations of medical practitioners in Huntingdon. The traditions of medical practice were changing as the roles of physician, surgeon and apothecary increasingly merged into the 'General Practitioner'.

The commercial challenge was to establish and grow a practice in the newly emerging 'medical market' in the town. Many new medical practitioners in the town and surrounding areas were in competition for funded public posts as Health Officials, and other salaried appointments such as in the workhouse or prison, factory surgeon and Friendly Society doctor. Such posts could provide regular income but required a network of contacts for recommendation and patronage.

To be successful in general practice with wealthier clients meant following codes of dress and social behaviour to gain respectability and social status. Appropriate marriage and family arrangements were advantageous. As Lady Warwick, the Victorian socialite, succinctly put it:

> 'Doctors and solicitors might be invited to garden parties though never, of course, to lunch or dinner.'[3]

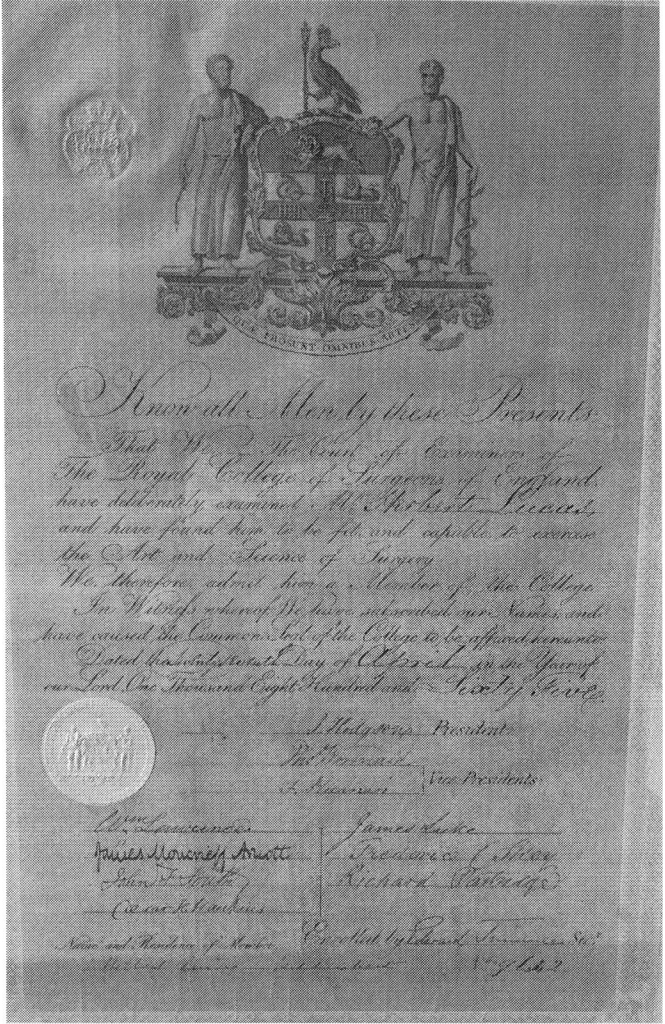

Certificate awarded to Herbert Lucas in 1865 following examination by the Royal College of Surgeons
(Charles Hicks Practice archive)

Medical work with the lower classes also continued, included treating ailments and diseases arising from poverty, poor housing, and continuing lack of sewers and drainage in some areas on the outskirts of towns such as Huntingdon and in nearby villages.[4] Improved transport such as increasing railway travel also enabled diseases such as tuberculosis, pneumonia and syphilis, to be more easily spread and cases continued to challenge practitioners even in rural areas.[5]

Personal life

The 1871 census records Lucas for the first time as a 'General Practitioner' with his practice based in High Street, Huntingdon. As a widower his life appears to have changed when he married for the second time in 1871, to Agnes Beart the eldest daughter of Robert Beart, Mayor of Godmanchester. Robert Beart was proprietor of Arlesey brick works who had won the contract to supply bricks to build the Town and

County Hospital in 1853.⁶ His brick works had already by this time made him wealthy as he had built 'The Chestnuts' in West Street, Godmanchester, described as,

> '....one of the best houses in the town. Robert Beart has expended a large sum of money in raising it and his gardens and pleasure-grounds, and in an embankment to exclude the floods.'⁷

Lucas's first known public post was obtained in 1876, when he was appointed a Councillor for Huntingdon. This was also the year that Michael Foster retired, and Lucas was able to purchase the High Street practice. He replaced Foster as Medical Officer at the Workhouse and Surgeon at the County Gaol, holding both posts for the next 10 years.

The Workhouse

The new Poor Law system was intended to be deliberately harsh with minimum comfort. People were given a basic diet and men and women were strictly separated. Husbands and wives lived apart, as did parents and children. The intention was to punish the 'work-shy' so that only the truly destitute or incapable would seek help. However, the Huntingdon workhouse was said to be one of the best in the country and provided three meals a day, rather better than many outside the workhouse enjoyed.⁸ As Medical Officer, Lucas would have been concerned that the workhouse drains and sewage facilities were the cause of much illness, such as unidentified 'fevers', probably including typhus, until they were improved following the Public Health Act of in 1875.

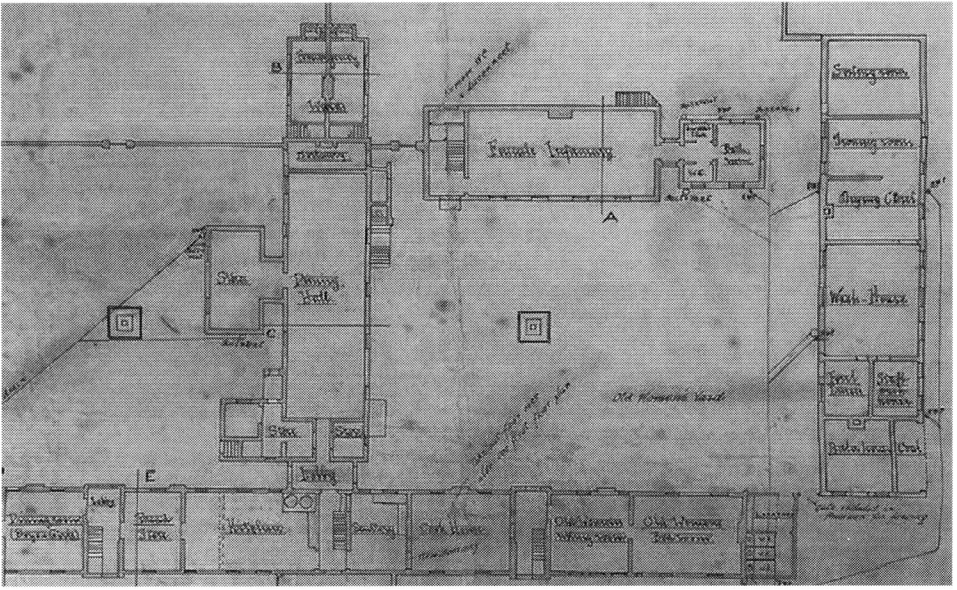

Plan of Huntingdon workhouse showing the female infirmary at the end of the 19th century.
(Courtesy Cambridgeshire archives)

The 1881 census for Huntingdon workhouse listed 169 workhouse inmates, of which there were 56 males, 40 females, 2 married couples and 62 children (listed as 'scholars'), with 7 babies and 5 staff. 73% of the men were aged over 60, the majority recorded as agricultural labourers. Only 33% of the women were over 60, with 40% listed as widows and 15% as single mothers.[9]

Being in a workhouse in 1881 was often a sign of desperate poverty, but it could result from several factors among them unemployment, old age, infirmity, and mischance in life events. There was little support for the poor in the community in the 1880s for mental illness and other disabilities. Asylums were intended only for those who could be cured or who were disruptive. This excluded *'harmless and incurable idiots'*, 10,000 of whom remained in the workhouses across England.'[10]

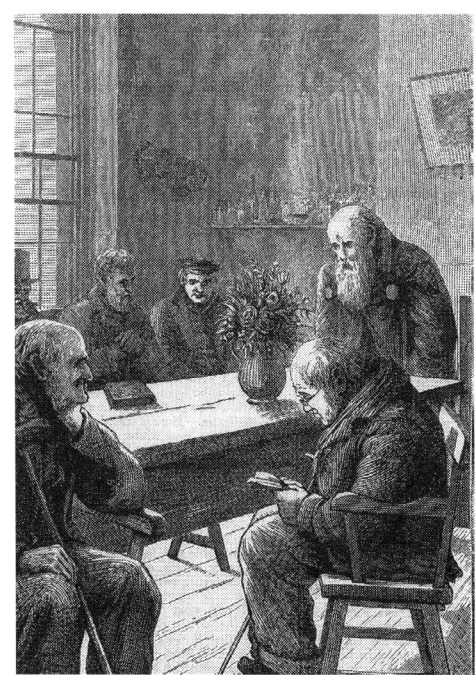

Old men in the workhouse
(Wellcome Collection)

The Asylum

The 'Three Counties Hospital' for Bedfordshire, Hertfordshire and Huntingdonshire was opened in 1860 on the site of the previous Lunatic Asylum in Bedford and 'fitted to the best standards of the day' and large enough to take a thousand 'patients.' This was a move away from previous treatment of 'restraint and bleeding' for those deemed 'insane' in the Asylum. The early rules at the 'Three Counties' stated,

> *'Bear in mind the insane are ill, and not responsible for what they say or do. They are sent to the asylum for their cure and to be taken care of. That they are afflicted and deserve our pity and consideration.'*[11]

At the Three Counties Hospital there was a library, gardens for growing vegetables, amateur theatricals and even a cricket pitch. However, there were still outbreaks of typhus, smallpox and influenza and an isolation building was erected in 1870. By 1885, records show that there had been 4,770 admitted, of which 1,800 had been 'restored to their friends' and 1,768 had died. A new water supply and drainage system was not introduced until 1904. The institution was renamed 'Fairfield Hospital' in 1960 and closed in 1999.[12]

Success in a growing medical market

Herbert Lucas became a respected medical practitioner among his peers. He joined the British Medical Association (BMA) in 1869 and was elected as President of Cambridge and Huntingdon BMA branch in 1881.[13] The census of that year shows him living at 108 Brampton Road with his wife Agnes, 4 sons and a daughter. The youngest son, Francis Clay Lucas was aged 3. The household also contained a governess and 3 servants. Private patients would still have been a major source of income at this stage of Lucas's career. Hard work was required, often involving travel at short notice and sometimes even overnight stays.

Nelson Hicks describes the GPs workload in his lecture on the History of Medicine:

"In the 1880s the GP was in the position of having to do the best he could with the material to hand. The run of the mill cases were the minor ones of injury to limbs, bad backs (lumbago hadn't been 'invented' until the 1900s), burns and scalds, varicose ulcers and tonsilitis. Epidemics arose at frequent intervals, and he had to be prepared for the loss of patients from diphtheria, scarlet (fever) and pneumonia for which the treatment continued to be a purge to start with, bed and hot bricks and febrifuge mixture standing by, with brandy and strychnine for the crisis and collapse on the 5th or 6th day."[14]

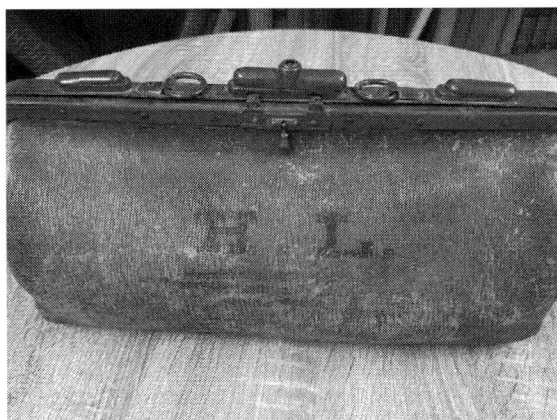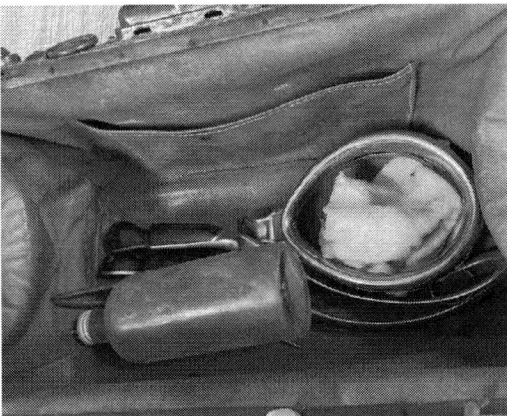

Herbert Lucas's medical bag and equipment, including forceps and chloroform pad.
(Charles Hicks Practice archive)

Home births continued to be another source of income. His BMA meetings exchanged information on current best practice and would have informed Lucas of the work of Ignaz Semmelweis, a gynaecologist in Austria in 1847, who had advocated hand washing and use of antiseptic procedures between examining women in labour. Semmelweis became known as the 'saviour of mothers' in demonstrating that washing hands and use of disinfectants could reduce the risk of spreading septicaemia. This went against medical opinion at the time, but by the 1870s, was beginning to be understood by medical practitioners in England.[15]

Improvements following the 1875 Public Health Act

The earlier Public Health Acts had been permissive, but in the 1860s and 1870s health policy expanded and aimed to prevent disease by reforming housing, sewage, drainage and water supply. All new houses had to provide running water and an internal drainage system. Refuse removal and sanitation projects were also begun in this decade, but although a Board of Health was established for Huntingdon, drainage and contaminated drinking water remained a problem.[16] The 1875 Public Health Act required the creation of the roles of Medical Officer of Health (MOH) to oversee local initiatives. At first these were GPs, but later doctors needed to have Diplomas in Public Health as well.[17]

The Medical Officer of Health had a higher public profile than a surgeon in the workhouse and Huntingdon gaol (which closed in 1895). The post was much sought after but Huntingdon and Godmanchester were slow to make appointments. In August 1875, a letter to the Board of Health from a Captain Roper stated,

"There is no Medical Officer of Health at the present time. Godmanchester has recently been visited by a very heavy flood the effect of which has been disastrous especially on the poor, whose cottages in one portion of the town have been left two or three feet under.......it is feared that it must in the end, result in some serious outbreak of fever. I know that the Union doctor, Mr Lucas is seriously alarmed at the danger."[18]

Herbert Lucas eventually became Medical Officer for Health and Public Vaccinator, but not until 20 years later, in both Godmanchester (1894) and then Huntingdon (1901). The annual payment for this role in 1890 was £30.[19] It involved collecting and analysing data to identify local sickness and mortality trends. Conducting inspections of drainage and poor sanitation which bred disease became important, as did encouraging hospitals to isolate those with infectious diseases.[20]

Huntingdon County Hospital

By 1890 Lucas had taken another important step in his career when he was appointed a Medical Officer at the County Hospital in Huntingdon. Working alongside him were Donald McRitchie and his brother David, who had established their own successful practice at 84 High Street, Huntingdon.

Dr Herbert Lucas (1863–1919) 33

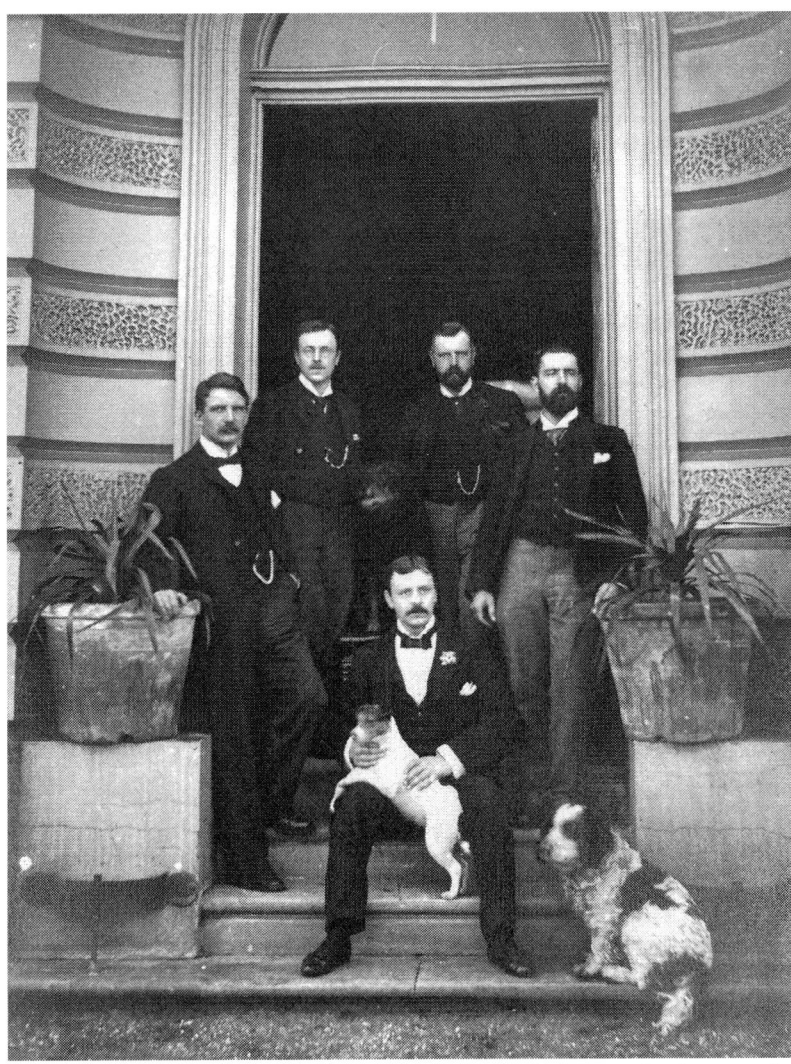

Herbert Lucas with Donald and David McRitchie and others at the old Huntingdon County Hospital in the 1890s
(Courtesy of Cambridgeshire Archives)

The Board of Management for Huntingdon County Hospital in 1888, noted: 228 patients treated, 1,006 out-patients treated, 105 visited in their homes. Inpatients still contributed only one shilling and sixpence per week. Huntingdon County was described as *'practically a free hospital'*.[21] The acceptance of private patients was recommended, with the first to be admitted paying 30 shillings per week, plus fees for their medical attendant.

In 1896, the Matron was Miss Barriman. She had trained as a nurse at St Thomas' Hospital in London and had been recommended by letter to the Board by Florence Nightingale herself.[22] Miss Barriman began a comprehensive training programme for nurses and upgraded their status, creating a separate role of 'Ward Maid' to wash floors and prepare meals etc. She was replaced by Miss Crawford in 1904, who was herself replaced as Matron by Miss Armitage in 1912 who did not finally retire until 1954 after 42 years of service to the County Hospital.[23]

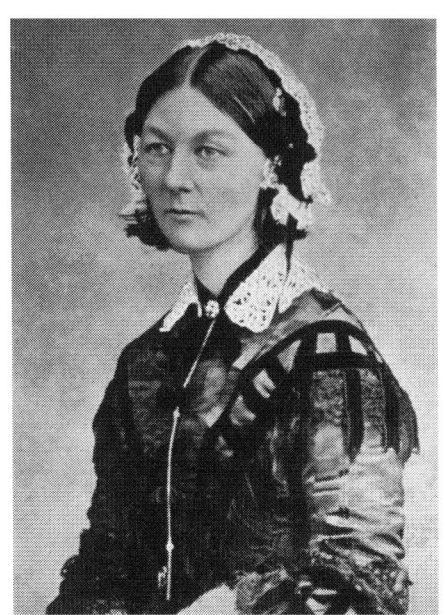

Florence Nightingale
(Wellcome Collection)

Florence Nightingale had established the world's first professional nursing school at St Thomas' Hospital in London, in 1860. Her 'Notes on Nursing' turned nursing into a respectable profession and would have taught Matron Barriman at the County Hospital, that hygiene, sanitation and cleanliness were crucial to the recovery of the sick.[24] An influential report by Matron Barriman in 1897, resulted donations successfully raising funds for the building of a new nurses' wing, an isolation ward, a new operating room and the re-flooring of all wards with teak floors to maintain cleanliness.[25]

In his surgical work at the hospital, Lucas would have seen significant improvements beyond cleanliness. By 1876, Joseph Lister had established the use of effective antiseptics (rather than carbolic acid) and soon after in 1881, Robert Koch introduced the sterilisation of instruments following surgery. Following the example of William Halstead in America in 1890, the wearing of surgical gloves during operations also soon became widespread.

By 1908 the sum of £130 had been approved by the Hospital Board for the purchase of a horse-drawn ambulance. It was kept in the coach house of the George Hotel which provided an attendant and a horse for two shillings a week. The attendant kept the ambulance washed, cleaned and oiled.[26]

The Isolation Hospital and Pest House

Lucas had been appointed as the Medical Officer at the Huntingdon Isolation Hospital in Primrose Lane, which was opened in 1898. It was a fever hospital and housed the elderly and people with contagious diseases. In 1914 there were 16 beds.

A mile further out of town (in a 'Pest House') there was a smallpox block with a further 12 beds.[27] The Pest House had been planned by Huntingdon Council and used since 1755 to house those with contagious disease such as smallpox or cholera. Lucas was responsible for the Sanitary Survey of 1893-5 which identified the Pest House with 5 beds at the time as 'very unsatisfactory.' The Pest House was eventually destroyed by fire in 1931.[28]

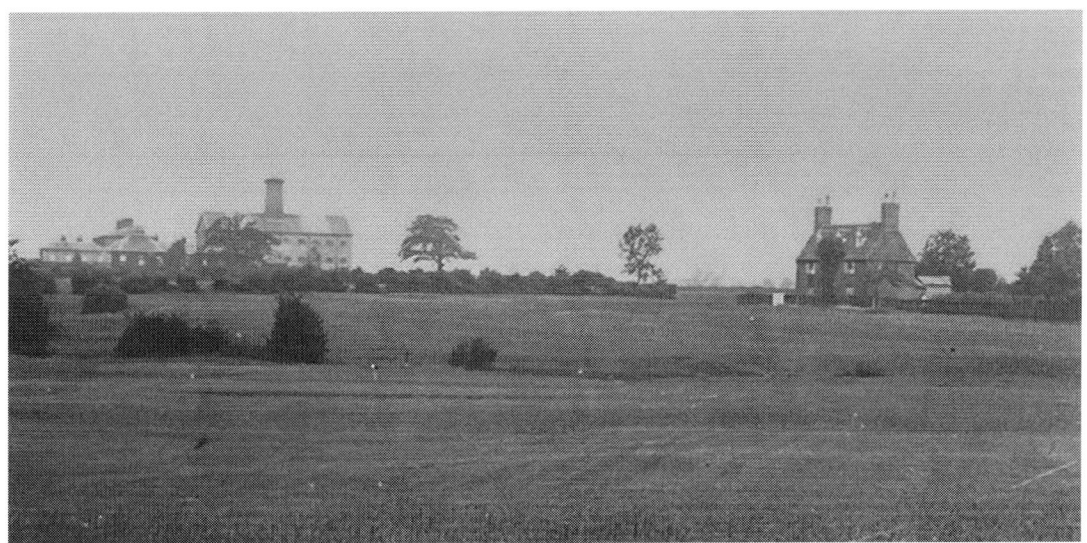

The Pest House on Spring Common with the County Gaol in St Peter's Road in the distance
(Courtesy of Cambridgeshire Archives)

Another event involving Herbert Lucas in 1898 and worthy of note, comes from 'Notes left by Revd Vicars', Parson of Little Stukeley, in December 1936.

"The bones of Joshua Slade who murdered the Revd. Joshua Waterhouse were bought from Mr Bryant of Cowper House, Huntingdon, by Dr Lucas in 1898. One of Lucas' assistants took some of them (an arm, I think) away with him when he left – but otherwise the skeleton is intact and now in the possession of Dr Hicks (Lucas' partner and successor)."[29]

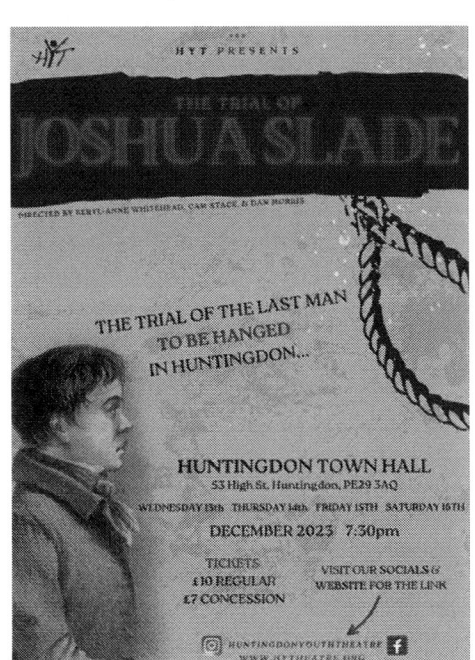

Poster for 'The Trial of Josha Slade'
(Patients' Forum archive)

Joshua Slade had been convicted of murder and was the last man to be hanged in Huntingdon, on Mill Common in September 1827. The whereabouts of the skeleton today remains unknown. A local Youth Theatre Company regularly recreates the trial in Huntingdon.

A new surgery at Bosworth House

In the 1901 census Lucas was living at 18 George Street, with Agnes, his daughter and 2 servants with a cook and a housemaid. In 1903, a major move took place as the practice expanded. Lucas moved his residence and practice to Bosworth House, a 19th century building at 157 Huntingdon High Street.[30] This was later to become the base of the Charles Hicks Practice until 1967 when the Huntingdon ring road was constructed.

The year 1903 was also significant as this was when Charles Hicks arrived as a newly qualified doctor in Huntingdon. He started work as assistant to the McRitchie brothers at 84 High Street.[31]

In 1911 the census recorded Lucas (age 68) still working as a surgeon, living with his wife and three servants. This was when Charles Hicks joined him as his assistant having left employment with the McRitchie brothers.

Lucas was still Medical Officer of Health for Godmanchester and Huntingdon Districts in 1914 (age 71).[32] Charles Hicks took over the practice in 1919 when Lucas eventually retired aged 76, and he probably passed his signed copy of 'Transactions' to Charles Hicks around this time.

Herbert Lucas died in 1922 leaving effects of £11,792 to two of his sons – Robert Beart Lucas (a manufacturer) and George Frederick Lucas (a solicitor). There is no mention in his will of Travis Clay Lucas, who moved to Chippenham after serving in the Army Medical Corps in WW1 and had become a farmer.

Other local medical practitioners

Donald Mc Ritchie

The father of the McRitchie brothers had been a chemist in Inverness, Scotland. Born in 1853, Donald had gained a Bachelor of Medicine Degree (MB) and Certified Midwife (CM) from Aberdeen and Licentiate of the Royal College of Surgeons (LRCS) from Edinburgh. He thus became the first qualified midwife in Huntingdon! Godmanchester records do not show a qualified female midwife until Mary Tester is named in 1911.[33] Donald McRitchie later became the Medical Officer for Health in Huntingdon district and Public Vaccinator for Huntingdon. He was also Deputy Coroner for East Huntingdonshire. He died in 1926 and is buried in Priory Road cemetery, Huntingdon.

David McRitchie

David was born in 1860. He gained Membership of the Royal College of Surgeons (MRCS) and a Licentiate of the Royal College of Physicians (LRCP) of London. He became police surgeon in Huntingdon. Just as Bosworth House became the centre of the Charles Hicks Practice in the 20th century, so the McRitchie practice at 84 High Street, Huntingdon, was to lay the foundations for the later practice, now on the ring road, known as Priory Fields.

Chapter 5

Dr Charles Hicks (1910–1948)
Foundations of the Charles Hicks Practice

"On opening the door (to Bosworth House) you went up the stairs and turned right into the waiting room and reported to a lady on reception at the far end of the room by the door that led to Dr Hicks' consulting room. The waiting room was dark and gloomy with pews along the back wall. When it was your turn the lady would call your name, hand you an envelope with your medical records and in you went."[1]

This account of a visit to Bosworth House at 157 Huntingdon High Street, is from a young patient in the 20th century and very different from attending either surgery of the Charles Hicks Practice today.

Dr Charles Hicks had his surgery at Bosworth House between 1911 and 1948. He provides an example of the classic 'general practitioner' in the communities of Huntingdon and Godmanchester through the significant events and medical developments of the early 20th century.

Training at Guy's Hospital Medical School

Born in 1874 in Tooley Street, London, Charles Hicks attended Guy's Hospital medical school in the 1890s, joining the Apothecaries Society in 1894. Guy's Hospital took increasing numbers of paying patients in their 14 wards at this time, and students had many opportunities to gain practical experience. Charles acted for 6 months as a 'Ward Clerk' whilst attending lectures in anatomy, physiology and the sciences, often also acting as a 'Dresser'[2] under supervision in the operating theatre.

Junior students attended maternity cases in patients' homes near the hospital (often at night). Charles Hicks' 'confinement book' shows that in one month (December 1898) he delivered 69 babies. A true 'baptism of fire' which set him up for his later practice in Huntingdon when, by his retirement, he had delivered at least 1250 children.[3] He also had training at Guy's in the treatment of infectious diseases at a Fever Hospital and possibly the two 'smallpox ships' moored in the Thames until 1903.[4]

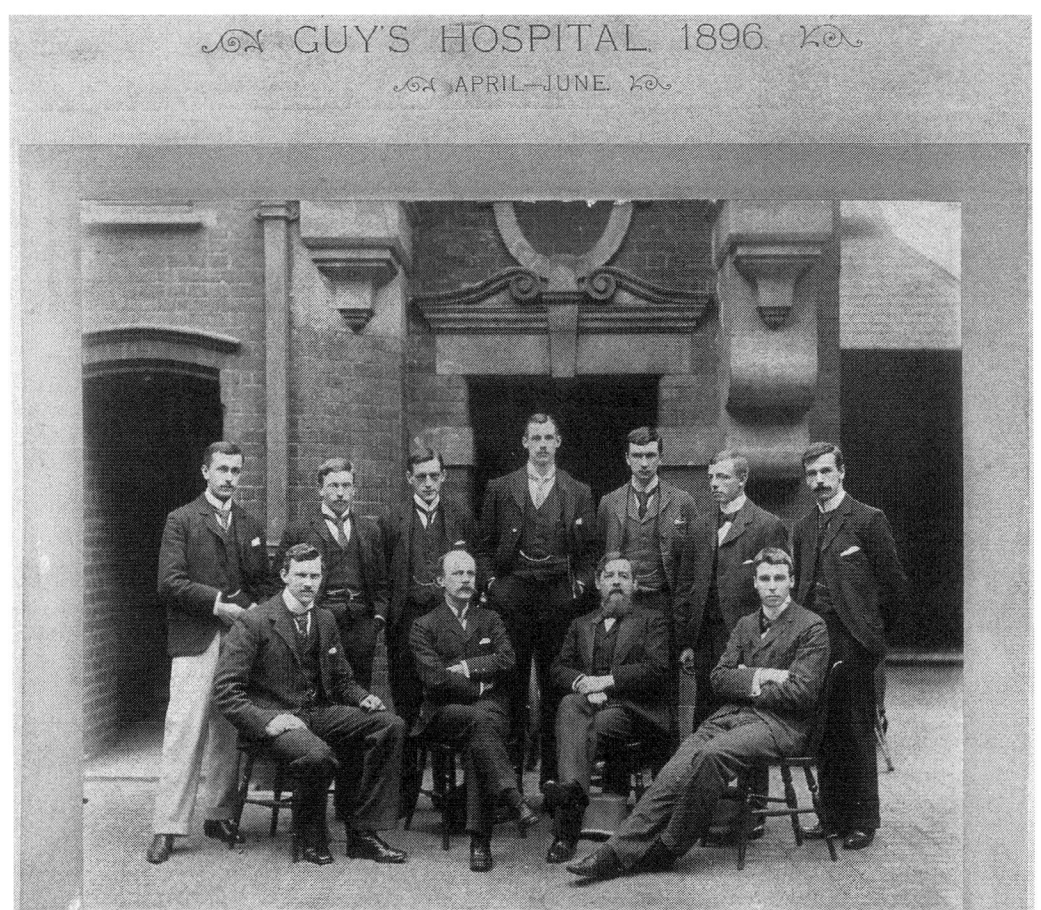
Sir James Frederic Goodhart with Lauriston Elgie Shaw and a group of students at Guy's Hospital in 1896 (Wellcome collection)

Charles passed his written and oral 'conjoint exams' from the Royal Colleges of Surgeons and Physicians covering anatomy and physiology, surgery, surgical anatomy and pathology, medicine and midwifery. His formal medical education and training had gained him the qualifications of Member of Royal College of Surgeons (MRCS) and Licentiate of College of Physicians (LRCP). However, as Reginald Grove, a contemporary who qualified from Guy's found, *"these qualifications were not geared for general practice life as they were largely designed for the needs of hospital medical specialists."* From a medical standpoint, general practice consisted of *"......a great deal of medicine, a fair amount of obstetrics and gynaecology and very little surgery, but the recently qualified man knows his work in the reverse order."* [5]

Arrival in Huntingdon

Recently qualified doctors needed to gain more practical experience in the community if they were to become successful in general practice. In 1901 Charles Hicks became an assistant at a well-established practice in Huntingdon with the

McRitchie brothers (see Chapter 4) whose practice was at 84 High Street. The 1901 census showed that Charles lived at 4 Sandringham Villas but later by 1903, he had married Grace and moved to 3 Hartford Road.⁶ Nelson Hicks their eldest son, was born the same year.

This busy practice would have given Charles Hicks a rapid introduction to the health and medical needs of the Huntingdonshire Community. Most women (95%) gave birth at home in 1905,⁷ and his confinement book shows continued deliveries of children (385 between 1901 and 1910) not only in Huntingdon and Godmanchester, but in Ramsey, Offord D'arcy and Abbots Ripton.⁸

Successful deliveries of home births were a way of building up fee paying clientele among the wealthier residents if the distance to travel was not too great. Registration of qualified midwives did not begin until the Midwives Act of 1902, so rural practices might use their assistant (usually male) if a doctor was called to attend a birth.⁹ Poor Law business also came to the practice as evidenced by 34 of Charles' recorded deliveries over this period being to women in the Workhouse. Not limiting himself to adult patients, in 1910 Charles Hicks was also appointed as 'Surgeon to the Boy Scouts' with a certificate signed by Baden Powell himself!

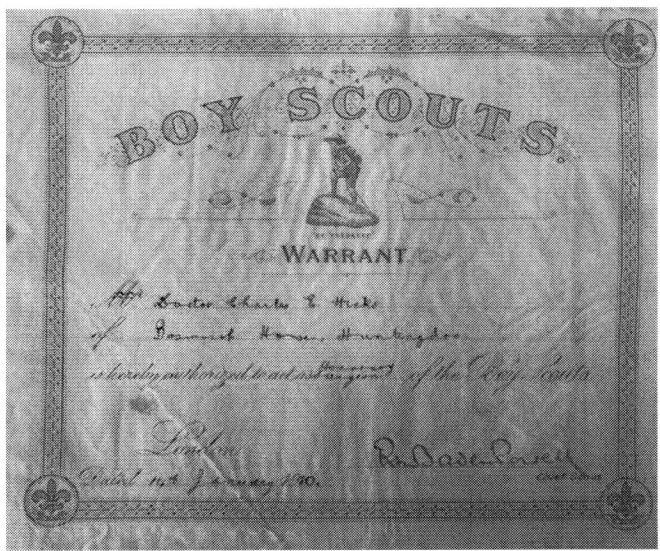

Certificate signed by Baden Powell
(Charles Hicks Practice archive)

In 1911, Charles joined the practice owned by Herbert Lucas, who was now 68 years old, still a practising surgeon living and working at Bosworth House at 157 Huntingdon High Street, with his wife Agnes, and 3 servants. In addition to his age, other reasons why Herbert Lucas might have sought an experienced assistant were not only the business opportunity afforded by the Liberal government's National Insurance Act of 1911, but also the increased administration that came with it. This Act gave participating 'panel doctors' a better rate of pay (7 shillings) per patient compared to many Friendly Societies, however record keeping in a standardised format was required. Records were kept in the famous 'Lloyd George' envelopes, and involved more administration than doctors in many practices were used to.¹⁰

The National Insurance Act of 1911

Throughout the 19th century working class men could mainly get access to a medical practitioner with fees paid through insurance schemes, usually run through Friendly Societies, unions or 'medical clubs.' However, insurance did not cover their wives, children or other dependants and there were very few 'benefit clubs' for working women.[11] In Huntingdon, Friendly Societies included the Ancient Order of Foresters, the Tuesday Night Friendly Society and the Manchester Unity of Old Fellows. Most prosperous, appears to have been the Lord Hinchingbrooke Friendly Society.[12] In Godmanchester, the 'Benefit Clubs' were smaller and less formalised. They were named after their meeting place and included the 'White Lion', 'Old Horseshoe' and 'Royal Oak'.[13] Membership nationally, peaked in 1900 when at least 50% of adult males in England paid contributions to such insurance schemes.[14]

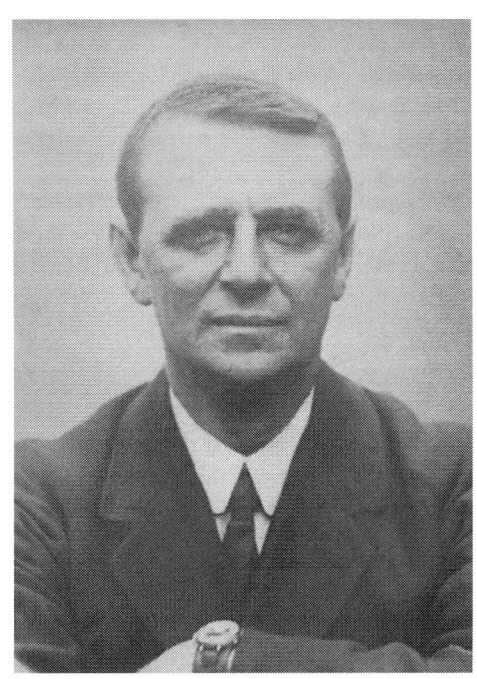
Charles Hicks
(Charles Hicks Practice archive)

The 1911 Act was based on the model of a national health insurance scheme set up in Germany in 1883. These schemes, which initially covered only the poorest workers, operated in the same way as private insurance, except that the workers' contributions were augmented by additional contributions from his employer and the state. The Act considerably weakened the role of Friendly Societies and clubs as the existing working class 'self-help' began to give way to state welfare provision for increased numbers of the local working population.[15] The Act set up a 'panel system' to approve treatment for patients who qualified, in order to be seen by the doctors who took part in the scheme. Most of these 'panel doctors' also kept on treating their private patients as well as any other public office duties.

A National Health Insurance Committee was based at 38 Huntingdon High Street, from which the local panel system for implementation of the Act was administered. We don't know whether Charles Hicks became a 'panel doctor' but most doctors eventually did. In Wisbech, there were riots when local doctors initially refused panel patients.[16] By 1918 over 16,000 general practitioners had signed up for contracts under the National Insurance scheme.[17]

The system excluded women and children, high earners and the self-employed. However, for working class men earning under £660 per year it provided, for the first time, free access to a 'general practice service', medicines and a small sickness payment. One consequence was the unexpected increase in the number of visits to the doctor. An estimate in *'Medical World'* in 1912 calculated that a panel practitioner saw 66% of their panel patients rather than the 30% that they had been expecting.[18]

The continued exclusion of women resulted in conditions left untreated by those who could not afford to pay. The journal *'Maternity Letters'* identified backache, neuralgia, varicose veins, headaches and prolapsed wombs.[19] Many of these were regarded with fatalism and continued to be treated with home remedies and over the counter medicines, as used by their mothers and grandmothers in the nineteenth century.[20] It was not until the start of the NHS in 1948, that this lack of access to medical care changed for most uninsured working class women.

Working at the County Hospital

In a more senior role with the Herbert Lucas practice, Charles Hicks was able to gain the posts and promotion that he would have expected. By 1912 he was appointed Honorary Surgeon at the County Hospital. His seniority was soon recognised, as it was recorded that '...*in May 1912, Dr John Morvatto was appointed House Surgeon at £100 per annum, with the proviso that Dr Hicks would countersign all his orders for drugs.*'[21]

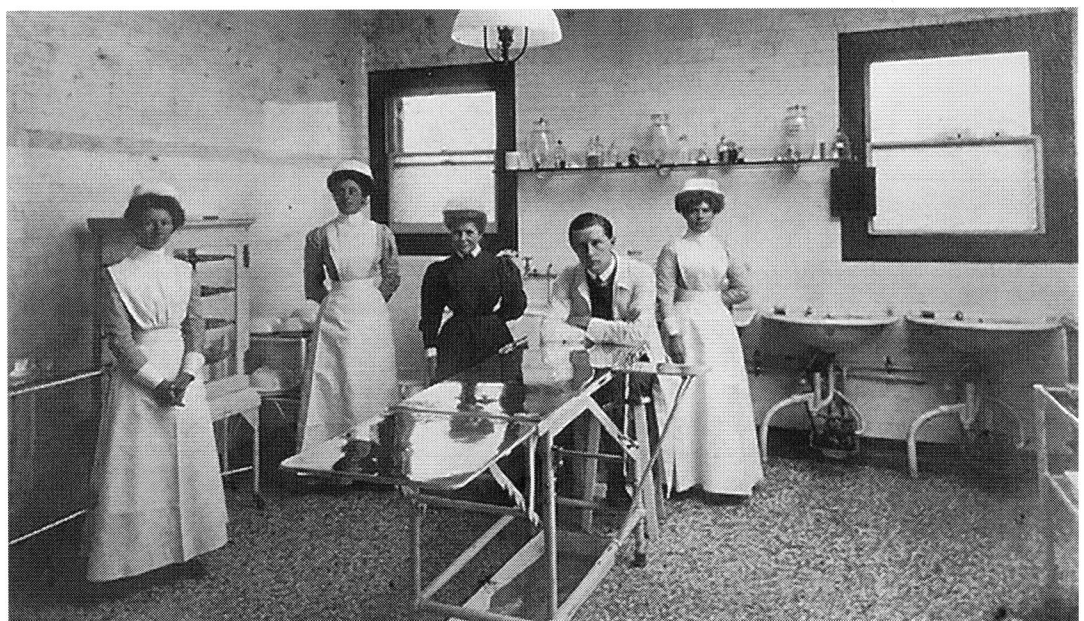

Charles Hicks in the operating theatre at the County Hospital in 1912
(Courtesy Cambridgeshire archives)

By 1914, the practice at Bosworth House had one of the first telephones in Huntingdon – the number was '38 Huntingdon'. The telephone exchange for the town was at Number 1 Priory Square, a small house just off St Germain St. Mrs Florence Saunders (mother of the mayor) operated the exchange in her front parlour.[22] This was known as the 'small telephone exchange'. It is said that Mrs Saunders *"probably took the first message to arrive in Huntingdon that Britain was at war with Germany."*[23]

World War One experience

In November 1914 the first fifteen wounded soldiers were transferred from Addenbrooke's Hospital to Huntingdon County Hospital. It was impossible to replace the House Surgeon (who had presumably joined the Army Medical Corps) with a qualified doctor and the unqualified substitute had to be supervised by honorary Medical Staff,[24] which would have included Charles Hicks. In March 1915 a relief hospital at Lawrence Court was also receiving the wounded.[25]

By December 1914, Walden House next to All Saints Church in Huntingdon, had become a Voluntary Aid Detachment (VAD) hospital with civilians providing nursing care for injured troops and other servicemen. Walden House was soon staffed by trainee Red Cross nurses under the management of Charles Hicks as Medical Officer, along with Miss Armitage, the Matron from the County Hospital and other ancillary staff. Walden House could accommodate 85 patients at a time until it closed in January 1919 – with 3,900 men having been treated – often as many as 50 per day.[26]

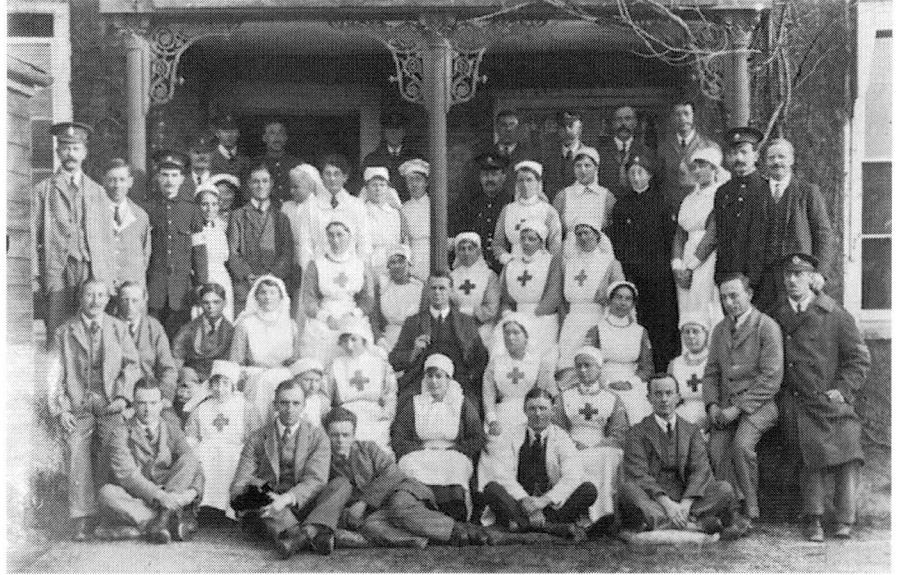

Charles Hicks with Red Cross nurses at Walden House in 1916
(Courtesy Cambridgeshire archives)

Despite his work at the County Hospital and Walden House (and the Boy Scouts), Charles Hicks was often the doctor 'on call' for births and medical emergencies. His 'Confinement Book'[27] shows that he assisted at 174 births during the war years. The *Hunts Post* shows reports of emergency 'call outs' during the war, many involving Godmanchester pedestrians (often children) being hit by speeding motorcycles.[28]

A more significant medical challenge for Charles Hicks towards the end of the war would have been to organise Red Cross nurses to cope with an epidemic of 'Spanish Flu'. First identified in Spain in May 1918, both soldiers at the front and civilians at home were struck down by a pandemic as

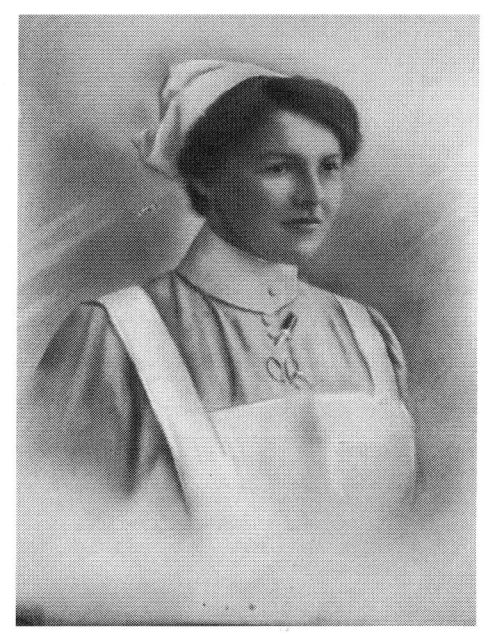

World War One nurse
(Charles Hicks Practice archive')

severe as COVID more recently. Over 5,000 British troops died and over 200,000 were taken ill.[29] Initial symptoms were like a common cold but could develop quickly into pneumonia with death often following in 24 hours. Attempts were made to limit social gathering and occasional mask wearing was observed. Despite many folk remedies being tried there was no known cure, but Aspirin tablets (which had been developed by Felix Hoffman, a German chemist working for Bayer) began to be used to relieve symptoms.[30] Also used was quinine powder dissolved in water, along with inhalers and vaporisers supplied by the Red Cross.

By the end of subsequent waves in the autumn of 1918 and May 1919, the death rate in the UK was at least 228,000,[31] and it was recognised that a national Ministry of Health needed to be set up in 1919 to better co-ordinate any subsequent pandemic.

In Huntingdon, deaths from Spanish flu can be estimated as at least 200, even allowing for the imprecise 'causes of death' recorded on many medical certificates. This represented between a quarter and a third of all deaths in Huntingdonshire in 1918.[32]

A new Practice is founded

After the war Herbert Lucas was seeking to retire. At the age of 76, he had kept the Practice going while Charles Hicks was employed at Walden House and the County Hospital. His son, Travis had returned from India and the Royal Army Medical Corps during the war, but records show no sign of him continuing to practice medicine. By 1922 the electoral roll shows that Travis was farming in Gloucestershire. In 1919 Herbert Lucas did retire and Charles Hicks took over the Practice and put his own name plate on Bosworth House.

Before the war Charles Hicks had taken over from Herbert Lucas as Medical Officer of Health for Huntingdon – a role which

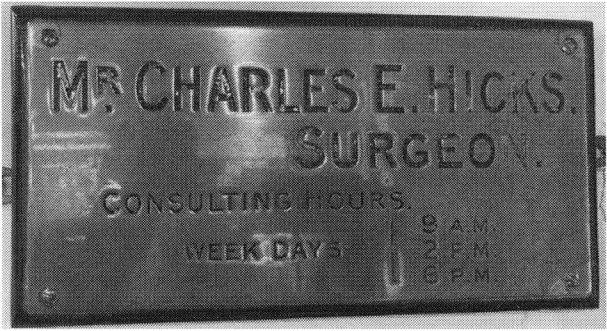

Charles Hicks Nameplate
(Charles Hicks Practice archive)

he performed for the next 35 years. He also had other public appointments such as County Hospital Honorary Surgeon, Medical Officer and Public Vaccinator for Godmanchester District, Certifying Factory Surgeon and Admiralty Surgeon.[33] Public appointments such as these had been important sources of income for Michael Foster and Herbert Lucas in establishing their positions as GPs in Huntingdon in the 19th Century and continued to be so for Charles Hicks.

A more unusual appointment for Charles Hicks was to be paid a retainer as Medical Officer to Huntingdon and Godmanchester Post Office providing medical care to the workforce. In 1914 the mail was collected 5 times a day and twice on Sunday in Godmanchester. There were three postal deliveries a day in the week and one on Sunday, so this was a very demanding job requiring high levels of fitness. The Medical Officer checked the fitness of new employees and treated injuries, ailments and sickness of staff.[34]

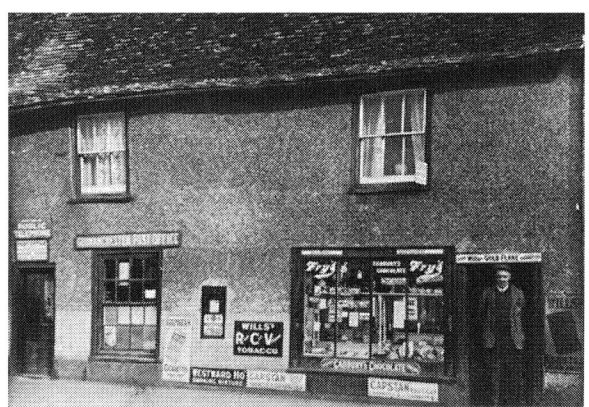

Godmanchester Post office in 1920
(Courtesy Cambridgeshire archives)

Charles Hicks was typical of single-handed practitioners in the inter-war years, so he could expect additional annual income from National Health Insurance 'panel payments' to make up between 25% -75% of his income.[35] The early demand for medical services from panel patients was unexpectedly high, partly as treatment was seen as 'free'. Also, working class male patients could now seek help at earlier stages of their illness and a 'sick note' from a doctor could be issued for the first time, ensuring payment of wages whilst unable to work. It was predicted that after 1911 there would be less than 2 panel patient-doctor contacts per year, but by 1931 the average nationally was 5 contacts annually.³⁶

His private patients (which did include women of the middle and upper classes) were important socially as well as economically. As Charles Hicks would have treated the whole community throughout Huntingdon and Godmanchester, he would certainly have been kept busy. The combined population of Huntingdon and Godmanchester in 1931 was 6,563 and there were only 2 main medical practices. He clearly undertook his work as a 'family doctor' with distinction for *'his friendly and cheerful manner, his painstaking care and attention, and his utter disregard of himself in the fulfilment of his duties of the profession of which he was such a distinguished member.'*³⁷

In the immediate years after the war, he did most of his home visits by bicycle.³⁸ He may also have gone on horseback or used a gig for some visits further afield.³⁹ Nelson Hicks later wrote of his father:

"If in the town, he had a brougham. In the country most of his near work was done on foot and his country visits were on horseback or in a gig or dogcart. Safety bicycles came later, and my father used nothing else for many years. He had surgery hours in morning, frequently three a day and three on Sunday. He was likely to be out for a good deal of the day, often having to stay the night at a patient's house if the weather was bad or the case was a difficult one. Of course, he was not bothered by telephones. Most messages were by hand or by courier." ⁴⁰

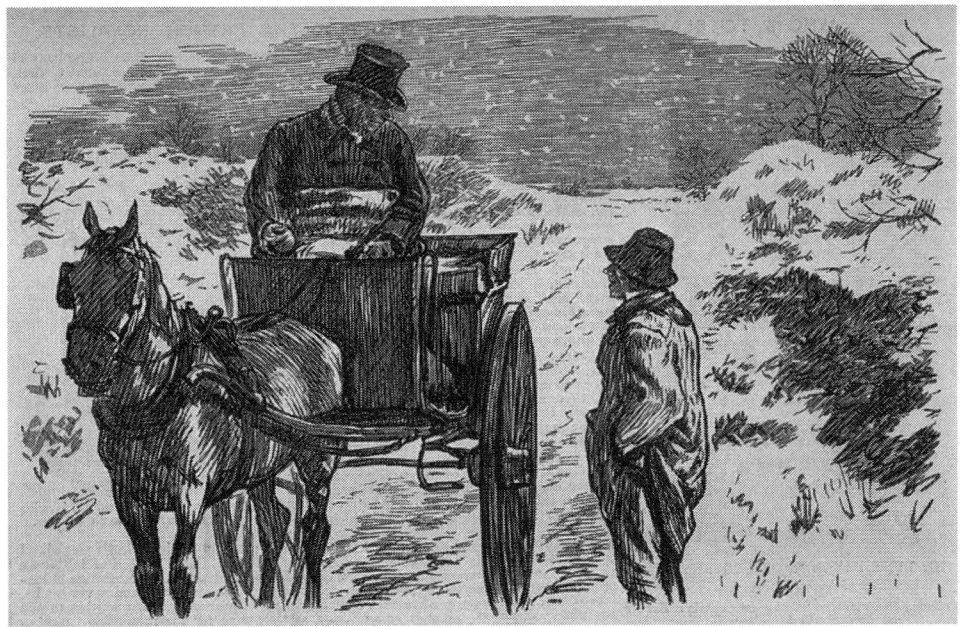

A country doctor asking for directions   (Wellcome Collection)

Public Health improvements

As Medical Officer of Health in the 1920s and 30s, Charles Hicks saw significant changes in public health with a new Ministry of Health having been established in 1919. This took over all local authority health-related provision such as midwifery and became responsible for all public health service provision. Interventions in public health and gradual improvements in standards of living slowly developed in the 1930s. For example, piped fresh water supplies were not installed in Huntingdon until 1935 and Godmanchester in 1936.[41]

One disease which persisted across the UK was the debilitating lung disease tuberculosis (TB), often linked to poverty and poor nutrition in the past, but also increasingly from occupational risks of working in crowded indoor environments in the first part of the 20th century. Although able to be better diagnosed with increasing use of X-rays in hospitals, TB often required many months of treatment and was still frequently fatal.[42]

The Cambridgeshire Tuberculosis (TB) Colony was an experimental scheme set up in 1916 by Dr Pendrill Varrier-Jones, the Cambridgeshire TB Officer, in Bourn. By 1918 it had moved to Papworth Hall and in 1929 the colony was renamed the Papworth Village Settlement, with new hospital buildings, and instruction in crafts and trades to encourage rehabilitation. Since 1921, the Public Health (Tuberculosis) Act had provided free treatments for all sufferers, even if they were not insured under the 1911 National Insurance Act.

Fresh air and light work were believed to be central to recovery (even in winter) and early photographs show patients' beds outside on balconies and others living in wooden shelters in the hospital's grounds.[43] Until the 1940s TB was the commonest cause of death in young adults.[44] It wasn't until the 1950s that tuberculosis began to be reduced with the development of antibiotics including Streptomycin in the 1940s followed with Isoniazid in the 1950s.[45]

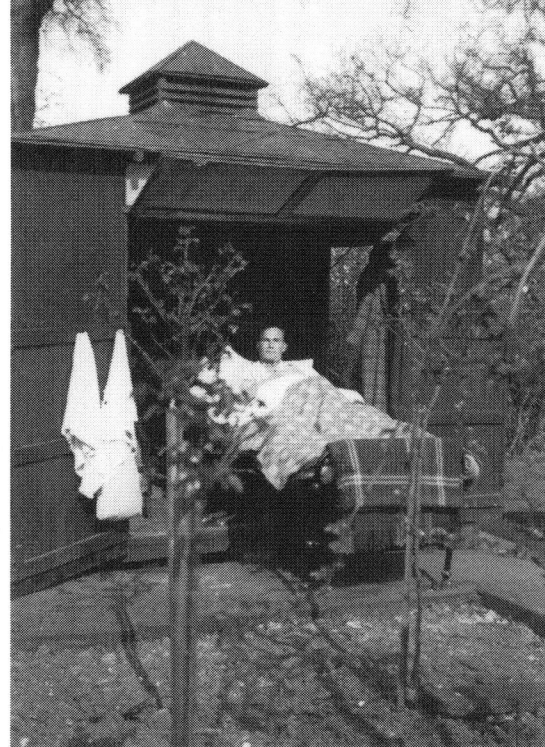

Henry Thompson at Papworth in the 1930s
(Courtesy Cambridgeshire archives)

A new partnership

Medical partnerships between GPs increased as demand for medical treatment grew and services expanded.[46] By the mid-1920s there was more work for the expanding Bosworth House Practice and Charles Hicks began a working relationship with Dr Peter Connan.

Peter Connan qualified as a doctor in 1924. He had assistant/locum posts in Alconbury and St Ives and then joined Donald McRitchie's practice at 84 High Street. He was also appointed as House Surgeon at the County Hospital and took over the High Street Practice after Donald McRitchie's death in 1926.

Peter Connan had been injured in his right leg at the battle of the Somme in WW1 and was recognised both as a skilled surgeon and an advocate for better public health. He eventually had his leg amputated in 1934 and continued to share patients with Charles Hicks whilst remaining at Number 84 Huntingdon High Street, establishing what was to become the Priory Fields Practice.[47]

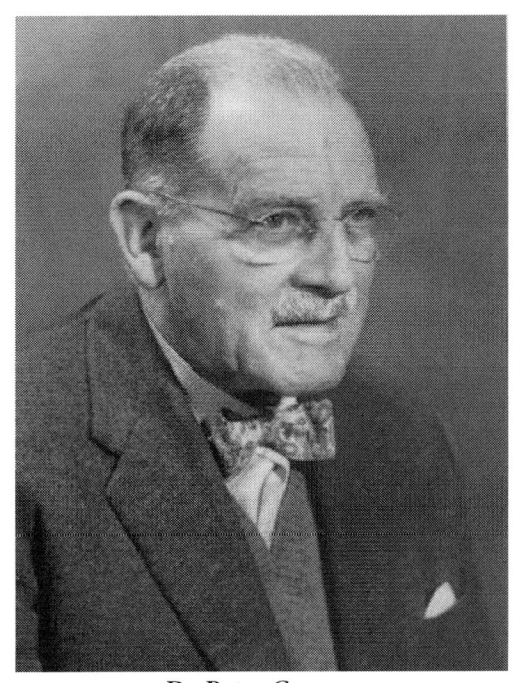

Dr Peter Connan
(Courtesy Dr Alex Connan)

Charles Hicks archives show evidence of a working relationship between Charles Hicks and Peter Connan, continuing right through the inter-war years, probably sharing a rota, and even sharing a jointly signed reference set of *'Illustrations of Regional Anatomy'*.

Supporting Peter Connan at this time, was the first female doctor in Huntingdon. His sister, Anne Connan had qualified as a doctor in 1923 and after working abroad, came to Huntingdon and lived at 84 High Street, working as a GP. She was also local deputy Medical Officer of Health and Assistant School Medical Officer.

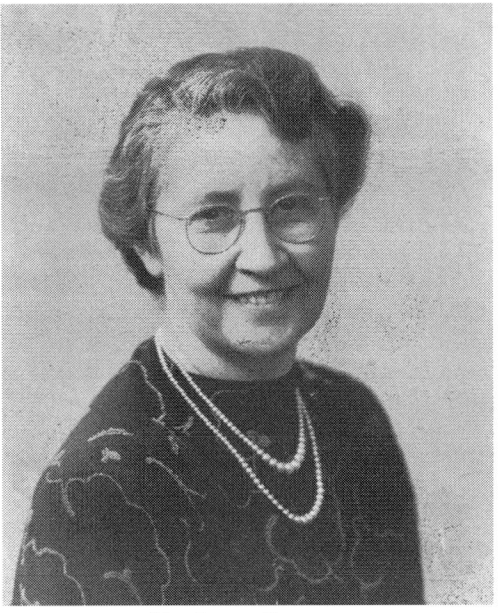

Dr Anne Connan
(Courtesy Dr Alex Connan)

Treatments and surgery

This inter-war period straddles the traditional and modern in medicine. Traditional medicine centred on diagnosis from observable symptoms and an interaction with the patient that could be close (if fee paying) or shorter for panel patients (when payment came from the state National Insurance system). A fifteen-year study of ailments in a typical rural practice like Huntingdon in the 1920s and 30s illustrates the workload for a single-handed GP. The study listed infectious diseases such as tuberculosis, diphtheria and scarlet fever in addition to TB. Childhood illnesses such as measles, chicken pox, whooping cough and mumps would also have kept both Charles Hicks and Peter Connan busy. In winter, colds, coughs and influenza increased for whole families, sometimes leading to bronchitis or pneumonia and in summer diarrhoea and typhoid.[48]

Advertisement for Mornay's Syrup
(Courtesy Cambridgeshire archives)

One commentator describes the role of the GP in the 1930s as follows:

'Successful treatment by the family doctor was accepted with gratitude and their many failures were tolerated with little rancour or recrimination. Patients' expectations were not high. Pain and discomfort were accepted as part of life to be endured with stoicism. The death of children from infectious disease was not uncommon. Treatments were still limited to thyroid extract, iron, digitalis, barbiturates, morphine derivatives and harmless mixtures. The advent in the 1930s of sulphonamides and then penicillin transformed the management of pneumonia.' [49]

The Charles Hicks archive has his Prescription Book. It was started in 1891 and handed down from Herbert Lucas on to Charles Hicks and later, on to Nelson Hicks (see Chapter 6). The first page is headed *'Solutions: Stock mixtures and ointments*

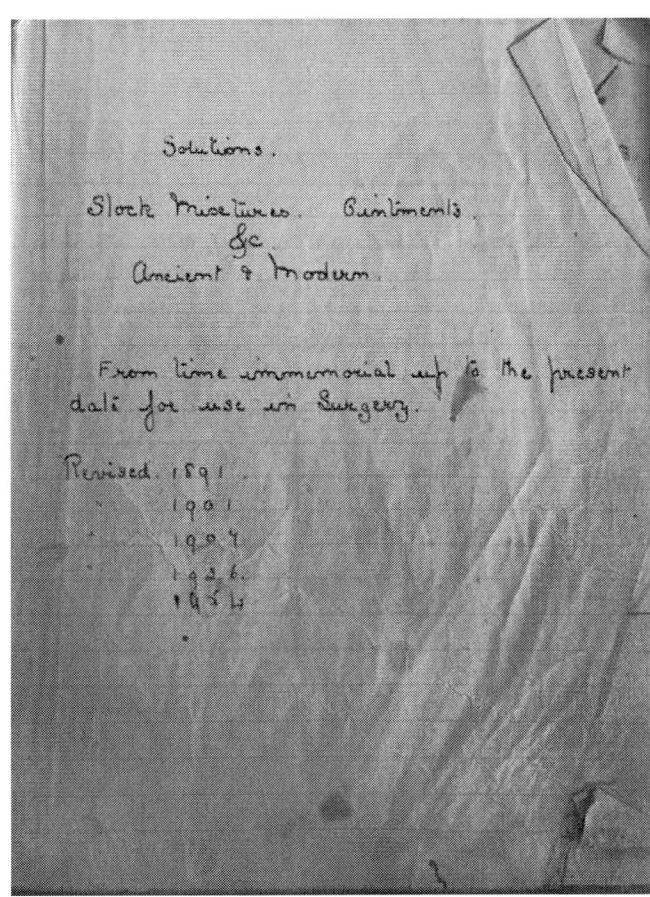
Prescription Book
(Charles Hicks Practice archive)

ancient and modern. From time immemorial up to the present date for use in surgery.' The Book shows that updates were added to the treatments used in 1901, 1907, 1926 and even up to 1954. Formulae used for individual prescriptions were a matter of professional pride and a doctor's 'special mixtures' continued to be an asset in building up a local reputation.[50]

By 1938, over 19,000 (75%) of GPs were National Insurance practitioners.[51] GP hours were long, as most practices were single-handed and deputising services were non-existent. A list of 2,000 patients was thought to be optimal size in rural areas, and a GP's wife often had a range of functions including the employment and supervision of ancillary staff. The role was pressured, combining the duties of receptionist, telephonist and secretary.[52] She was often crucial to the practice's success which could not otherwise be run safely and efficiently. Grace was Charles Hicks' lifelong companion and partner and her part in his success should not be overlooked. See also Appendix 2.

Medical advances

Modern medicine began to rely more on measurement using instruments, pharmaceutical intervention and referral to hospital when necessary.[53] Charles Hicks and Peter Connan represent the 'old school' GP who had a duty of care to patients and their families over their lifetime, whilst willing to adopt new equipment and techniques as required. New equipment included a microscope, stethoscope, testing equipment for urine samples and blood pressure as well as instruments for minor surgery.[54]

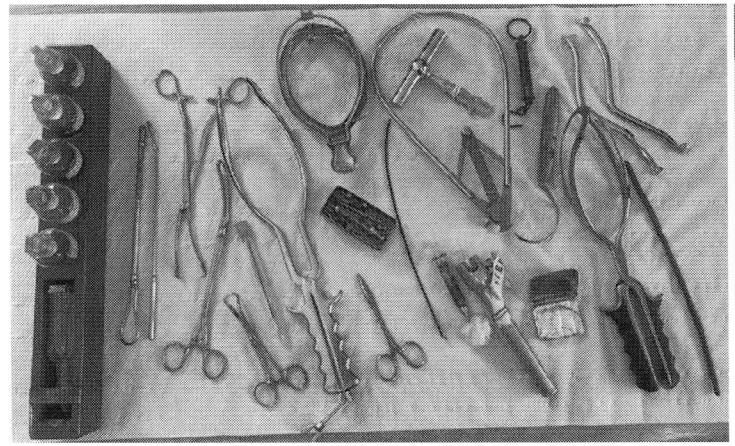
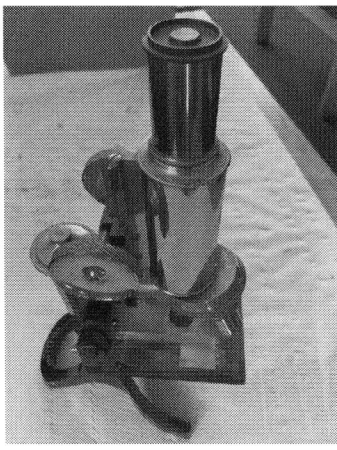

Charles Hicks' microscope and medical instruments
(Charles Hicks Practice archive)

The 'Story of Huntingdon County Hospital' shows that Dr Greenwood of Godmanchester had been appointed as Radiologist in 1927. Charles Hicks had a hand in supporting such 'modern' developments. In 1930, the Hospital minutes show that Dr Hicks had *'made proposals to the Board for improvements to the x-ray and massage departments, an anaesthetic room and a surgeon's changing room. These were agreed.'*[55]

In addition to working with Peter Connan and Anne Connan at the County Hospital, other doctors in Huntingdon over this period with whom Charles associated included:

Dr Jesse Garrood (1874 -1959) who was a GP in Alconbury between 1899 and 1958. He was Medical Officer of Health for Huntingdon Rural District (1924 -1958) and Public Vaccinator for Alconbury, Sawtry and the Giddings District. During WW1 he had served with the Huntingdonshire Cyclist Battalion in France.

After WW1, Dr Garrood had his Practice in Alconbury. *'He ran his surgery from a small green painted building that was little more than a garden shed. It is recalled that the surgery was so small that you had to stand outside in a queue to see the doctor, yet in this building Dr Garrood saw his patients, prescribed, dispensed medicines, and even did operations such as removing tonsils.'*[56] This surgery building later became the pavilion for Alconbury Weston Cricket Club!

Dr Veitch of St Neots was a member of the staff at the County Hospital between 1924 and 1948. He was *'always a very popular figure – especially with the nursing staff'.*[57] In 1928, he was appointed as an 'eye specialist' but also carried out Caesarian Sections when required. *'A very versatile man!'*[58]

Midwifery became a declining source of income for many GPs as the Midwives Act of 1936 encouraged more professional training and a gradual decline in home

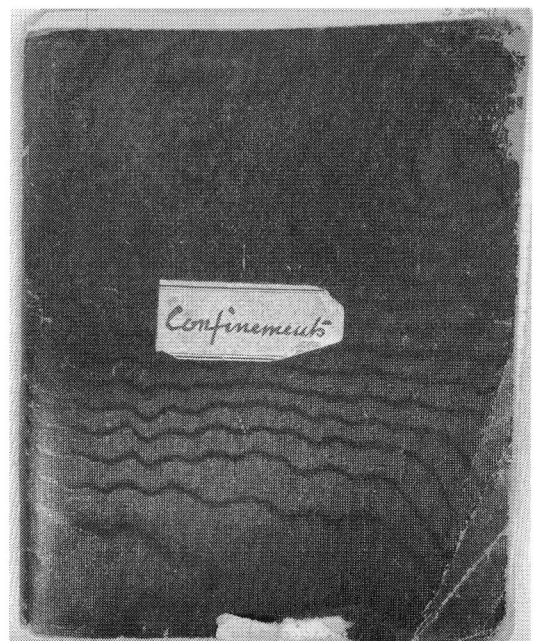

Confinement book
(Courtesy Cambridgeshire archives)

births nationally during the inter-war years. The first mentions we have of midwives in Godmanchester are Mary Tester in 1911 and Emily Springthorpe in 1920.[59] Charles Hicks' 'Confinement Book' still has records of home deliveries through to 1945, but these decline in number to single figures during the 1930s.[60]

World War Two

Charles Hicks continued to live in Bosworth house with his wife, Grace. His household at this time included a medical dispenser called Estelle Purnall, along with Hannah Rosamond (a cook aged 55), Margaret Cooper (a housemaid aged 20) and Mabel Denny (a widowed housewife aged 69). Mrs Pink had the rest of Bosworth House as a nursing home.[61]

By this date Charles's eldest son Nelson Hicks had qualified as a doctor and was becoming established in his first Practice on the Isle of Sheppey.

From 1939 to 1945 the Huntingdon County Hospital Records Book shows both Charles Hicks and Peter Connan still working together as they are among the doctors listed as visiting the wards, as was Dr Anne Connan. Other doctors listed are Dr Jolly, Dr Greenwood, Dr Veitch, Dr Grave and Mr Roderick (surgeon).[62]

Hicks and Connan also probably collaborated during the war in other ways as anecdotal evidence suggests that Peter Connan kept a cow to provide fresh milk, whilst Charles Hicks started to keep hens at Bosworth house to ensure a supply of eggs.[63]

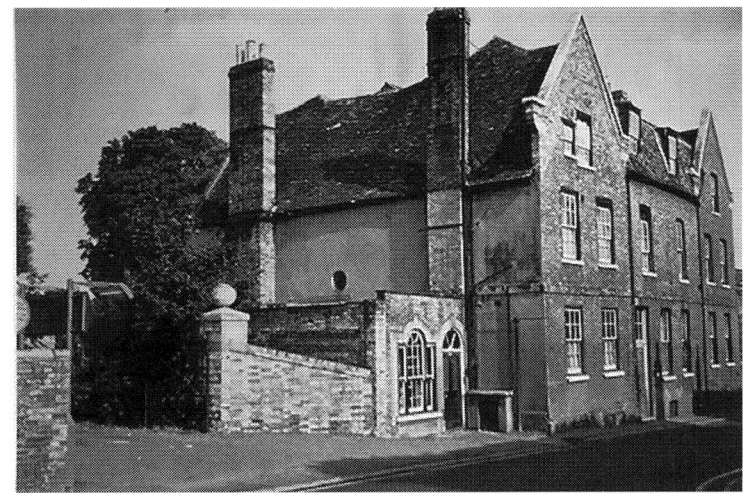

Bosworth House at 157, Huntingdon High Street
(Charles Hicks Practice archive)

First-hand accounts

It is from the 1940's that we get the first glimpse of Charles Hicks with first-hand accounts from patients who met him as young children, and whose comments probably reflect the imposing experience of *'being seen by the doctor.'* In 1944, John Thackray (then aged 5 or 6) had a chest infection, possibly tuberculosis. Charles Hicks was called for a home visit and ultimately referred him to a specialist and a stay in a London hospital. John now remembers him as *'quite a grumpy sort of bloke.'*[64]

Another patient was Danny Reid, who was evacuated to Huntingdon in 1941 as result of the Blitz. His mother registered Danny and his brother (born in 1939) with Dr Peter Connan's practice at 84 High Street. Aged seven, and with Dr Connan not available, Danny was taken to Bosworth House to be seen by Charles Hicks as he needed treatment for *'boils on both knees'* that his mother was unable to lance herself.

Going up some dark stairs to the waiting room with medicine bottles around the walls could be an alarming experience for a child. Dr Hicks, who is remembered as rather austere, referred Danny to the Town and County Hospital. The hospital doctors treated the boils – but also took the opportunity to keep Danny in hospital and have his tonsils taken out! Danny fondly remembers the red dressing gown that the hospital gave him to wear as some consolation.[65] See Appendix 3 for more on Danny Reid's story.

The end of an era and the beginning of the NHS

Charles Hicks reverted to working as a 'sole practitioner' after the war. Despite the 'heavy calls' made on him by his medical work, Dr Hicks found time for the pursuit of one of his favourite hobbies – the study of bird life in the county. He was remembered as *"……an expert in this subject and to discuss with him his wonderful collection of British birds' eggs or to share his enthusiasm over the hitherto unknown visitant to the Fens or the reeds by the Ouse was an unforgettable experience."*[66] We also know that he was interested in local history as in 1934 he signed his personal copy of Robert Fox's 'History of Godmanchester, published in 1831 and he also had a personal signed copy of 'The History of Huntingdon' published in 1824.[67]

Dr Hicks was a frequent visitor at Walnut Tree House (the old Workhouse) where he was known to the elderly residents as 'Uncle Charley'. To those who were very ill the knowledge that he was coming could be a big step towards recovery and to those who were convalescing his visits were awaited with pleasure. For many years he acted as 'presiding genius' and Father Christmas at the Christmas dinners.[68]

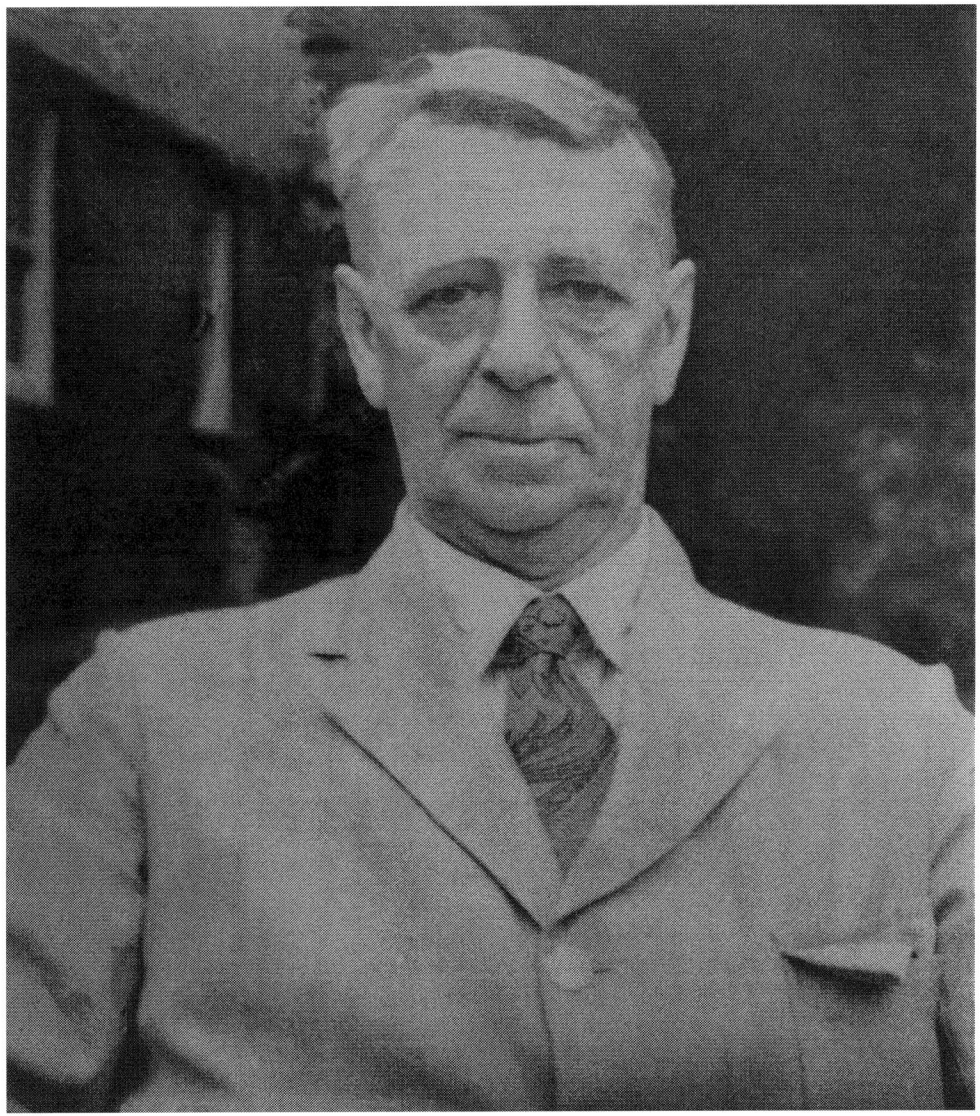

An elderly GP – Charles Hicks in the 1940s
(Charles Hicks Practice archive)

Times in the medical profession were changing and Charles Hicks was by now in his 70s. In 1947, Nelson Hicks joined his father at the Bosworth House Practice, having returned to Huntingdon with his wife Lavender, from a practice in the Isle of Sheppey.

Charles Hicks retired in 1948 having handed over the Practice and his copy of 'Transactions', together with the potential of a new NHS contract, to Nelson Hicks. He died aged 77 whist in London to see the coronation of Queen Elizabeth. Charles Hicks' funeral was held in St Mary's Church, Huntingdon with a large congregation made up of his family, professional colleagues, Huntingdon Freemasons, plus friends and ex-patients. Among the professional colleagues were Dr Garrood from

Huntingdon and Dr Hynes from Godmanchester, along with staff from the County Hospital, the Isolation Hospital and the Woodlands Old Peoples' home (including Mrs Pink from Bosworth House) and the Godmanchester Derby and Joan club.

In Chapter 6, we turn to the first of our doctors where his son, Nelson Hicks, took over the family Practice.

In 1948, Charles Hicks wrote a letter to Nelson Hicks outlining some of the issues that could be expected to arise as a GP in the community. This is his concluding paragraph in his own handwriting and below as a typescript in the archives at the Practice.

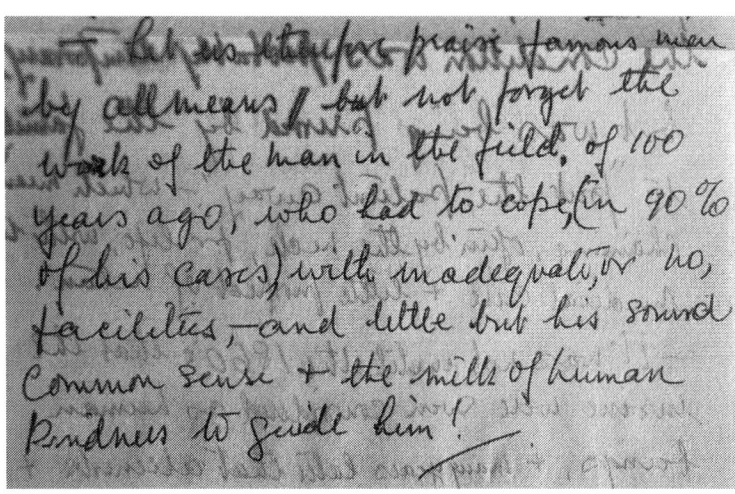

Let us therefore praise famous men by all means but not forget the work of the man in the ~~file~~ field, of 100 years ago, who had to cope, (in 90% of his cases) with inadequate or no facilities, and little but his sound common sense and the milk of human kindness to guide him!

Another GP in Godmanchester

Athur Atkins Greenwood was born in Islington, London, in 1886 and qualified as a doctor in January 1909. He undertook various roles at Guy's Hospital and then became Medical Officer in charge of the X-Ray department at Hampstead General Hospital. In WW1 he volunteered as a radiologist and went to France with the British Red Cross. He later joined the Royal Army Medical Corps and was posted to Serbia, where he worked in the 37th General Hospital in Salonika. He was awarded the French Croix de Guerre and the Serbian Order of St Sava.

After the war, Arthur Greenwood returned to general practice in London. He moved to Godmanchester in 1925 and lived in Fox House on Post Street (later to be the surgery for Dr Hynes). Greenwood worked as a GP in Godmanchester until 1946. In 1927 he was also appointed Honorary Medical Officer and Radiologist to Huntingdon County Hospital, where he worked with Charles Hicks and Peter Connan.

He retired from his hospital role in 1951, aged 65 and emigrated to Kenya with his wife and daughter. There he took charge of the X-ray department at the Nakuru War Memorial Hospital. Arthur Greenwood died in Mombasa in 1978. [69]

Chapter 6

Dr Nelson Hicks (1947–1973)
Following in his father's footsteps

"He was born in Huntingdon, where his father was the doctor. As a small boy he used to help his father in the surgery, holding bowls and passing instruments, so it was inevitable that he would join the profession." [1]

Dr Mike Whitton sets the scene for the only father to son transition in the Hicks Group Practice. What do we know about Nelson Hicks who continued to manage the 'Charles Hicks Practice' through the first 25 years of the National Health Service?

Training and first Practice in Kent

Nelson Hicks was born in Huntingdon in 1903. After attending Epsom College, he qualified from Guy's Hospital medical school like his father and in 1927, gained Membership of the Royal College of Surgeons (MRCS) and Licentiate of the Royal College of Physicians (LRCP). He was a member of the 'Innominate Club' at Guy's, a dining and debating society for medical practitioners. He loved motorcycles and once claimed that he rode from Guy's in London to Bosworth House in Huntingdon without touching the handlebars! A rather unlikely story?[2]

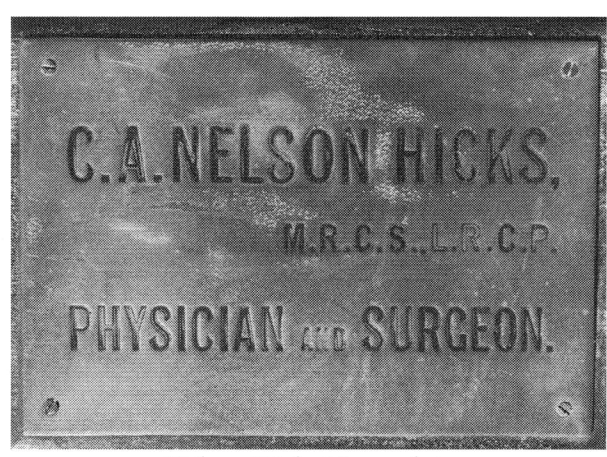

Nelson Hicks Nameplate
(Charles Hicks Practice archive)

In 1927, Nelson Hicks moved to the Isle of Sheppey for his first GP Practice, with his wife Lavender, whom he married the same year. Nelson Hicks became well-known for riding a horse when doing his rounds. On his return to Huntingdon, he rode with the Fitzwilliam Hunt until the late 1970s, and was course doctor to Huntingdon Steeplechase.

By 1947, Charles Hicks (then aged 73) needed support with

Bosworth House Practice and Nelson returned as his partner, taking on the Practice and with it the new NHS contract, in 1948.

Nelson and Lavender initially lived in the flats at Petersfield Hospital and later in St Peter's Road, Huntingdon.

The beginning of the NHS

Preparations for the National Health Service (NHS) were underway at the end of World War 2 with the election of a Labour government and Aneurin (Nye) Bevan as Minister for Health. In the NHS Act of 1946, Bevan planned a tripartite system of nationalised hospitals, GPs and local authorities. There would be 20 hospital boards (with some pay beds), GPs as independent contractors, supported by local authorities for community health, vaccinations and midwifery. Many GPs, led by the British Medical Association (BMA) representing 75% doctors, were not in favour as they feared 'state control', the loss of independence, their income from private patients and other contracts.

By 1948 a compromise had been reached. GPs retained the right to continue as independent self-employed practices and, like hospital consultants, were given a pay increase linked to the number of their patients if they were contracted through the NHS. Pharmacists, dentists and opticians in England and Wales also agreed to join the NHS.[3]

On 5th July 1948 the NHS began, taking control of 480,000 hospital beds, 125,000 nurses and 5,000 hospital consultants. Around 85% of GPs elected to join the new service. A leaflet was sent to every household in England and Wales assuring people that the NHS would,

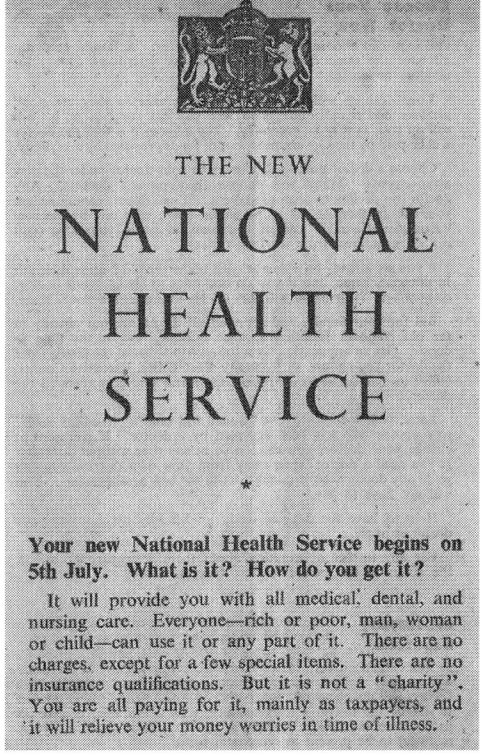

> '...provide you with all medical, dental and nursing care. Everyone – rich and poor, man, woman or child – can use it or any part of it. There are no charges, except for a few special items. There are no insurance qualifications. But it is not a 'charity'. You are all paying for it, mainly as taxpayers, and it will relieve your money worries in time of illness.'[4]

(Wellcome Collection)

For the first time, health care, free at the point of delivery, was extended from insured working class men to the whole population. Workloads in practices like Nelson Hicks at Bosworth House, rose considerably with untreated illness soon appearing – especially women who had suffered for years with chronic conditions.[5]

Paperwork changed: bills were no longer necessary but there were forms for eye tests, sickness certificates and milk rations. The entire registered population had an NHS 'brown envelope' with their medical records. These were transferred from one GP to another when they moved, along with GPs notes, vaccination information and hospital letters.

Initially, many GPs were overwhelmed. Pay per patient was only 20% above the level of 1939, until pay rates were raised again in 1952. Charges for dentures and spectacles for adults were introduced in 1951 by a Conservative government as the NHS budget escalated. Adult prescription charges were also added in 1952: one shilling for prescriptions and £1 for dental treatment.[6]

A single-handed GP in Huntingdon

By 1952, there were 17,000 GPs in the NHS with 1,600 assistants and 300 trainees. Half were in partnerships but in rural/semi-rural areas at least a third were like Nelson Hicks, single-handed, with patient list sizes limited to 3,500.[7] The combined population of Huntingdon and Godmanchester in 1951 was 7,784.

A report by Joseph Collings in *The Lancet* in 1950 was based on 55 General Practices outside London. Collings found *'no capacity in waiting rooms, no couches and poor record keeping'*. He concluded that *'there are no real standards for general practice. What a doctor does and how he does it, depends almost wholly on his own conscience.*[8] This report was followed by further studies, leading ultimately to the foundation of the College of General Practitioners in 1952.

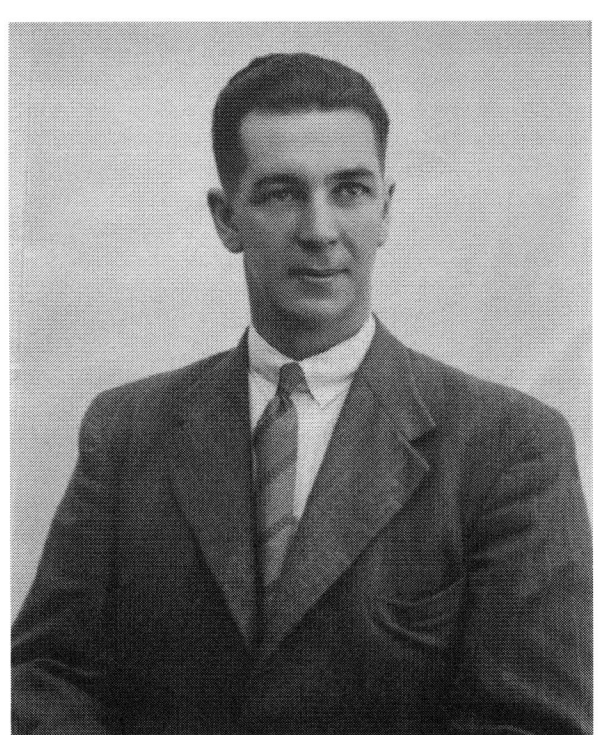

A young Nelson Hicks
(Charles Hicks Practice archive)

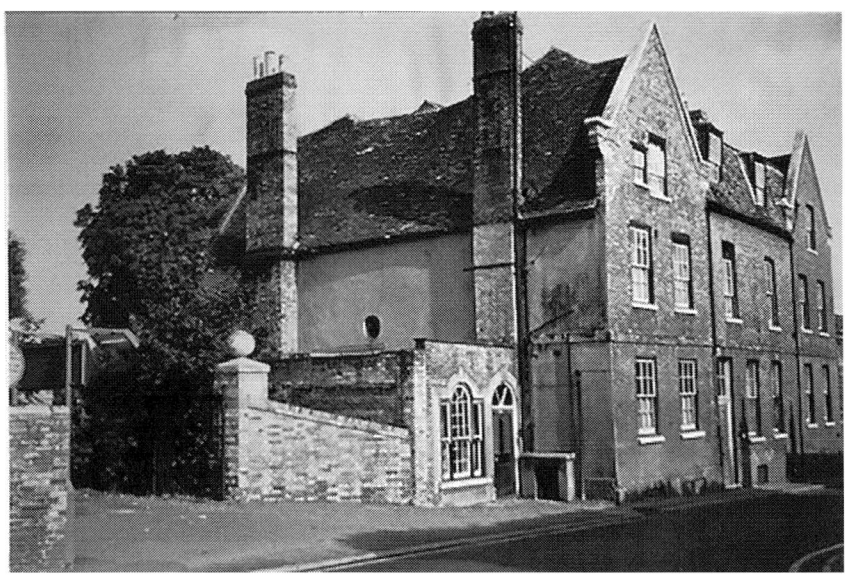

Bosworth House
(Charles Hicks Practice archive)

This view of rather eccentric working conditions is supported by comments from some of Nelson Hicks' patients at the time. Robert Picking recalls,

"On entering the consulting room, Dr Hicks was sat at a desk with his back to the window. You sat down and he attended you. To his left was a tall glass cabinet with medical instruments laid out, next to it was an old teddy bear from his childhood. On the other side of the room was an examination couch covered with a black oilcloth material on which you lay if needed."[9]

Robert continues,

"Bronchitis, Measles, Chickenpox, stitched cuts, bashed heads were all treated in that room. A room with a layer of blue tobacco smoke hovering about two feet from the ceiling. Dr Hicks smoked Capstan full-strength untipped cigarettes."[10]

Pat Roberts also highlights Nelson's smoking habit:

"I remember him as a real 'no-nonsense' man. He was bluff and straight to the point, no small talk. If my memory serves me well, I remember him sitting in his surgery, quite a dark room with a big desk. He always had a cigarette alight and as a young person I was always a bit scared of him. His receptionist was lovely though, I think her name was Alice."[11]

These rather intimidating views of Nelson Hicks from the childhood memories of patients can be countered with stories of his teddy bear. Nelson and his wife Lavender did not have any children and Nelson's childhood teddy, with the addition

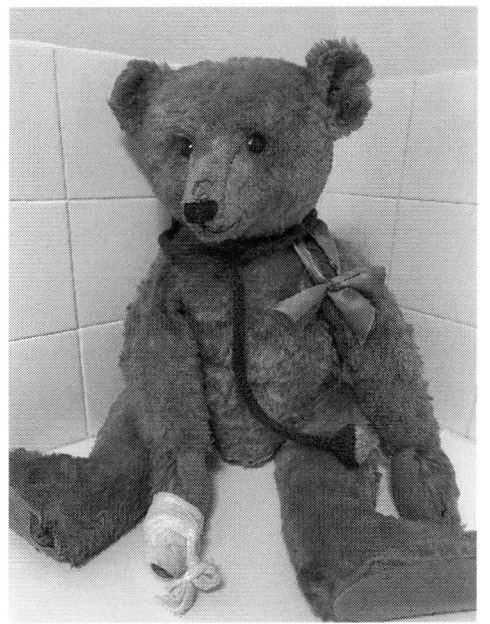

Teddy bear belonging to Nelson Hicks
(Charles Hicks Practice archive)

of bandages and knotted stethoscope, was kept in his surgery to placate younger children or to 'show where the hurt was'. The same teddy is still in use in the Roman Gate surgery to this day!

Home births

Not all Nelson's patients came to the Bosworth House surgery. *'Home births were the norm and his log of these extends to several hundred'*.[12] No longer on horseback, Nelson Hicks now had a succession of cars for home visits. Each had the registration number WOT 5 transferred to it. Senior and retired midwives all told stories of him sitting in his car after each successful delivery, smoking cigarettes and watching the sunrise.[13] He typified the level of care that followed from living in a small community.

John Thackray says, *"There were few ante-natal classes at first, so mothers were very reliant on their doctor."*[14] He goes on to say of Nelson Hicks (nicknamed 'Jim' by his friends) *"He delivered all our four sons. In 1967, our third son was delivered at home in mid-winter. As the midwife was late arriving, 'Jim' and Dr Rushden (also Jim) came – but both wearing pyjamas under their coats!"*[15]

For all sole practitioners, as Charles Hicks had found, the provision of 24-hour cover was problematic as well as finding cover for holidays and leisure time. District nurses and midwives were now employed through the NHS.[16] Nelson's childbirth responsibilities were supported in 1956 with the arrival of Doreen Mart (Nurse Mart) in Godmanchester, which must have provided some relief. She lived in the nurse's house in Post Street and then Windsor Road. She delivered them as babies and subsequently treated many Godmanchester residents when they became adults.[17]

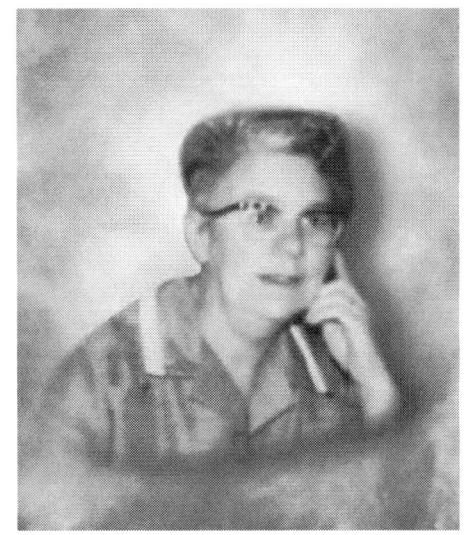

District nurse Doreen Mart
(Courtesy Verna Hayes)

Rita Day says,

"I can remember nurse Mart coming round in her little mini car with a big black bag on the back seat. My two younger sisters were both born at home in Hilsdens Drive. I thought my new baby sisters came out of that bag."[18]

Doctor Hynes in Godmanchester

Other doctors shared lists in Godmanchester (as Charles Hicks and Dr Connan had previously done in Huntingdon). Dr Hynes had a Practice in Post Street, Godmanchester from the early 1950s. He ran a baby clinic and dispensed tasty biscuits as well as Jelly Tots to the children.[19]

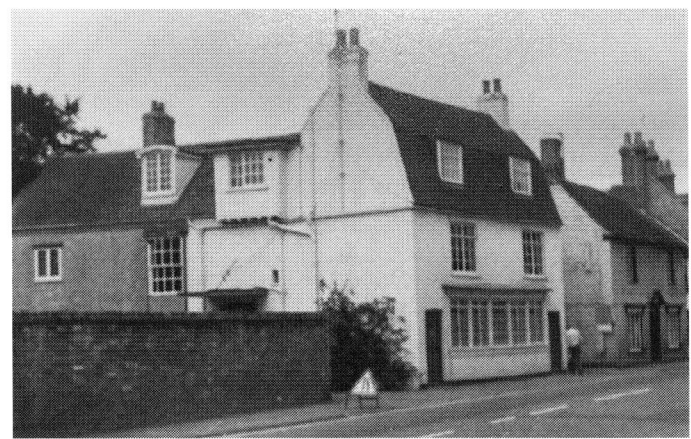

Dr Hynes surgery at Fox House in Post Street
(Courtesy Cambridgeshire archives)

Many Godmanchester residents, including Les Williams, Jules Barrell and Tony Dighton, remember him very fondly:

"Dr Hynes was a lovely, friendly man and my doctor as a tot," "I got a bead stuck up my nose when I was five, he got it out and gave me a Jelly Tot for being brave. He was such a lovely man", and *"Johnny Hynes looked after us all. You could ring him up in the middle of the night and he would always come out."*[20]

Clive Parcell also recalls,

"When a lorry carrying bottles of whisky lost its load on Horseshoe Bend, I heard Dr Hynes was outside his surgery encouraging patients to help themselves as it was better than any medicine he could give."[21]

Doreen Mart worked closely with Dr Hynes. She was a midwife for many home births in Godmanchester, Huntingdon and surrounding villages and RAF bases up the mid-1960s. She also ran ante-natal clinics at Nursery Road, Huntingdon, as well as post-natal visits, along with home dressings, injections, blood samples and support with other minor ailments. She shared her list with two other local District Nurses – Nurse Moate and Nurse Meeks ('The 3 Ms').[22]

The District Nurses worked with local doctors to administer immunisation programmes for the most infectious childhood diseases. By 1956, vaccination programmes were in place for smallpox, whooping cough and diphtheria. Later a live polio vaccine was developed and many children of the early 1960s remember having this administered by a nurse on a sugar cube. This was followed in 1968, by an effective and safe vaccination to protect against measles.[23]

Doreen Mart worked with Dr Middlemiss after 1969 and later Dr Gupta. From the 1970s onwards Doreen led the Godmanchester Brownies and Girl Guides. She was also a Quaker elder, with meetings based in the old Rose and Crown pub.

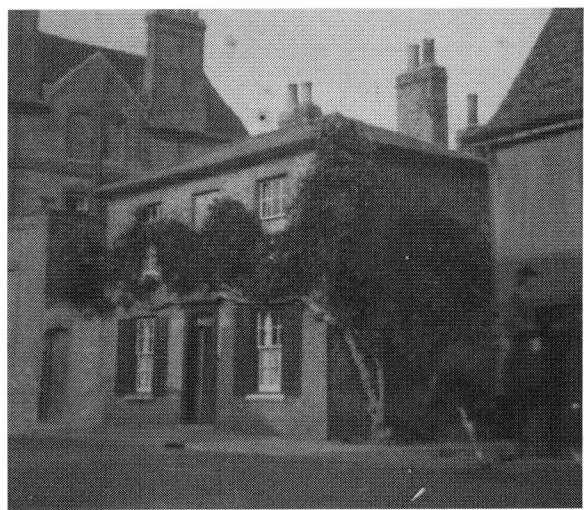

Nurse Mart's house in Post Street
(Courtesy Verna Hayes)

New ailments and new treatments

Therapeutic advances throughout the 1950s were extending the range of conditions that family doctors could manage effectively. Vaccines, steroids, antibiotics and other drugs continued to arrive. A shift in patterns of illness was underway as social and economic advances impacted on improved health. An extension for Outpatients was added to the County Hospital in 1955. Doctors like Nelson Hicks began to see less infectious disease and more degenerative diseases with the ageing of the population.

Big pharmaceutical companies like ICI, Glaxo, Wellcome and Beechams produced new drugs such as synthetic penicillin to treat sepsis and infection, blood pressure tablets and vaccines for tuberculosis, polio, whooping cough and diphtheria.[24] The costs of drugs prescribed by GPs grew quickly. Nevertheless, the 1956 Guillebaud Enquiry showed that the NHS cost overall was still falling as a percentage of Gross Domestic Product.[25] The Conservative, Enoch Powell later became Health Minister and raised prescription charges to two shillings to cover a proportion of these costs in 1963.[26]

The Bosworth House Practice began to treat more long-term chronic diseases like diabetes, with screening, blood testing and health promotions. The GP role was changing from treatment of infections and minor illness to more complex chronic disease management and prevention.[27] This presumably included the 'stop smoking campaign' and could explain the leaflet for a Portable Ozonizer in the Charles Hicks archives. This device was reputed to disguise the smell of cigarettes. For Nelson

Hicks this would probably have been an essential piece of equipment in his surgery.

Staff increases

More clinical and health care resources at the Practice were increasingly required and in 1961, Nelson Hicks recruited Ernest David Falla MRCS, LRCP as an assistant who was also an anaesthetist. Soon the Practice further expanded when Martin Pritchard, a recently qualified Batchelor of Medicine (MB) from Cambridge University, joined. Dr Falla was widely known as 'Dr Fellows' as described by Robert Picking:

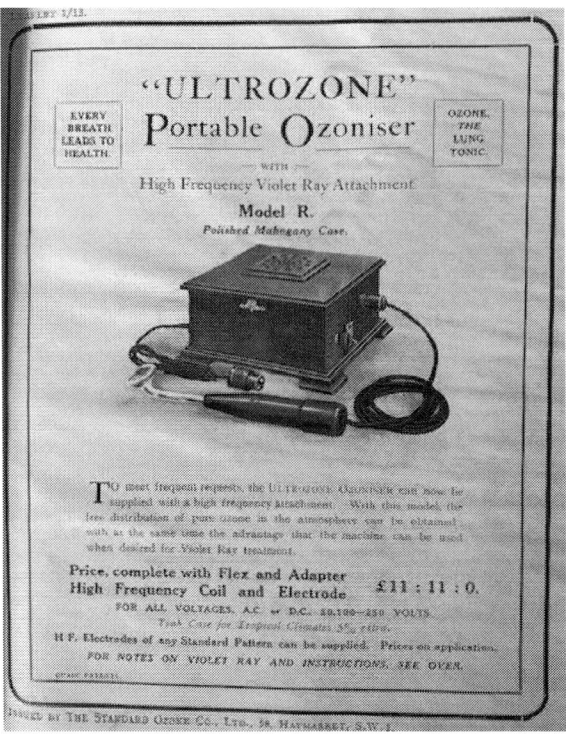

Portable Ozoniser leaflet
(Charles Hicks Practice archive)

> "Dr Fellows joined the Practice mid-1960s. In those days the doctors made home visits. Dr Fellows was frequent visitor to attend me and my siblings' ailments. He seemed a big man with a bald head."[28]

Changes were also underway in the other Huntingdon Practice at 84 High Street. Dr Peter Connan retired in 1960 and his partner in the Practice, Dr 'Bunny' Forbes, was joined by Peter's son, Dr 'Dan' Connan. That Practice expanded as well, with Dr Derek Cracknell leaving the RAF to join them. Later he established the MAGPAS air ambulance service. Dr Sibthorpe and Dr Phillips were also to join that Practice in the next few years. Also, as Dr Alex Connan remembers,

> "Dr William Love, an obstetrician, became GP and provided very skilled extra support with GP maternity cover at Primrose Lane Hospital."[29]

Big changes at Bosworth House

Two developments in the mid-1960s laid the foundations for the Charles Hicks Practice we know today. The first is the appointment of a new assistant and later partner, Dr 'Jim' Rushton in 1965. The second is the compulsory purchase of Bosworth House in 1968 to demolish it and make way for the new Huntingdon ring road. Nelson Hicks fought a long but unsuccessful battle to retain his lease on Bosworth House and prevent its demolition.[30]

The search for new premises eventually ended with the move to a much smaller converted bungalow at 19 Temple Close, Huntingdon. Despite the smaller premises in the *"tatty old bungalow"* as Wendy Stukins, a member of staff described the new premises,[31] the new energy and enthusiasm of Dr Rushton could not have come at a better time. Nurse Eileen May joined the Practice soon after the move to Temple Close, having been 'headhunted' from her role as Ward Sister at the County Hospital by Dr Rushton.

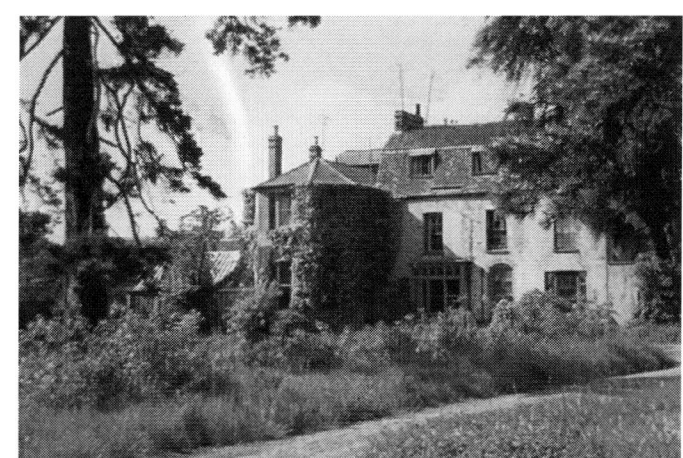

Rear view of Bosworth House
(Charles Hicks Practice archive)

A family doctor charter

In 1966, the 'Family Doctor Charter' had been introduced by the new Labour government. A new contract with GPs gave a pay increase to reflect increasing workload, skills and responsibilities. Doctors were also reimbursed for 70% wage costs for up to two nurses and ancillary staff in expanding practices. The NHS budget now also covered the costs for vaccinations and cervical smears as part of the move towards 'anticipatory health care'.[32]

Nelson Hicks was well known and respected in both Godmanchester and Huntingdon. He had become a core member of the community. As Dr Keith Stewart describes him,

> *"Dr Nelson" was a General Practitioner of the 'old school': he would not tolerate malingerers but won the greatest affection of the patients who genuinely needed him. He was a gentleman to a fault, a smart dresser and lively wit"*[33]

Bill Adams remembered him as,

> *"Every Christmas morning he would visit Huntingdon Police Station with two big tins of homemade mince pies and a few bottles of spirits for the officers on duty that day,"*[34]

and from Rosemary Lemmon,

> "Dr Hicks came to me when Dr Hynes was on holiday. He always carried a jar of home-made toffee for the children, which would be frowned upon these days."[35]

Nelson's role as course doctor to the Huntingdon Steeplechase continued after his retirement in 1973 and he also remained keen on shooting throughout his life. John Thackray remembers Nelson Hicks going clay pigeon shooting with his father,[36] and Bill Adams says,

> "I had dealings with Dr Hicks in the disposal of his many varied firearms as in later years, he wandered round his garden shooting rabbits with a military revolver."[37]

Nelson Hicks continued to work as a locum for the practice until 1977. He and Lavender retired to Hunstanton where they were visited by many friends and old patients. Dr Keith Stewart writes,

> "His health was failing but he was always pleased to have company and his wit was with him until the end."[38]

Nelson Hicks died in 1983. However, the Charles Hicks Practice had been born and continued to develop and meet new challenges under the excellent leadership of Dr Jim Rushton (see Chapter 7).

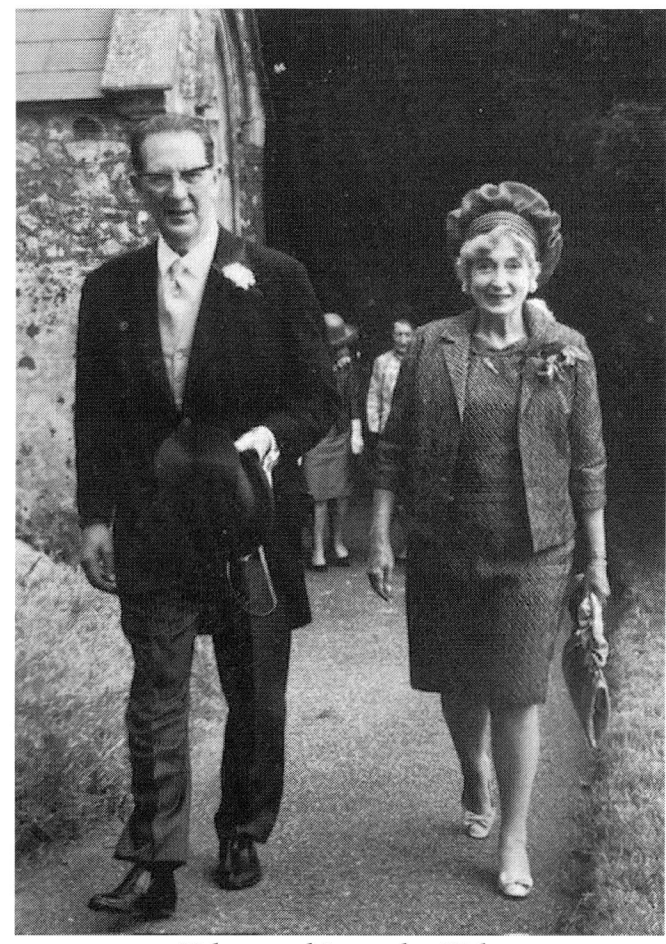

Nelson and Lavender Hicks
(Charles Hicks Practice archive)

Chapter 7

Jim Rushton (1965–1995)
Formation of the Hicks Group Practice

"I found his loyal patients truly appreciated his calm competence and brief, accurate and to-the-point diagnostic, explanations. He was invariably right, and patients got better as he expected. He was not an enthusiast for flattery, either given or received. One was competent (or not). "Well done, boy" was as good as it got, and one knew then that one had lived up to his high standards."[1]

Dr Keith Stewart's picture of 'Uncle Jim' Rushton gives an overview of the man behind the development of the Hicks Group Practice as we know it today.

Early Years

Jim Rushton was born in Chingford, Essex in 1932 but evacuated to Stoke on Trent in 1939 staying with his grandparents. In 1949 he won an Open Scholarship to Kings College, Cambridge to study medicine, graduating in 1956 as a Bachelor of Medicine and Surgery (MB, BChir). In 1957 he undertook clinical training at the London Hospital, Whitechapel, gathering Diplomas in Anaesthetics and Obstetrics and Gynaecology. He also gained Membership of the Royal College of Surgeons (MRCS) as well as a Licentiate of the Royal College of Physicians (LRCP).

Dr Rushton started as a house officer at the London Hospital, Whitechapel. In 1965 he moved to Huntingdon where he became junior partner with Dr Nelson Hicks in Bosworth House, also working part of his time as an anaesthetist at Moffat's the dentist in Huntingdon.

At the Charles Hicks Practice, he oversaw the increase in the number of doctors to eight on his retirement, with the creation of three surgeries in Huntingdon and Godmanchester as well as at RAF Wyton. He played a very large part in the formation of

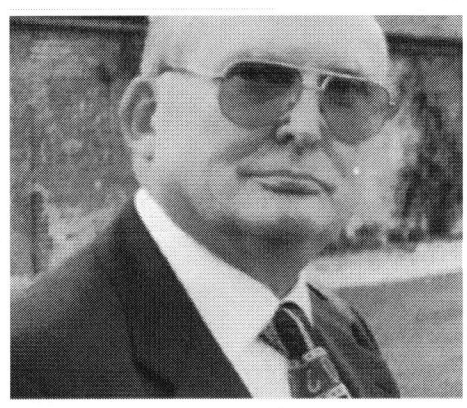

Dr Jim Rushton
(Courtesy of the Hunts Post)

what is now called the Hicks' Group Practice. He was known to the support staff throughout his time at the Practice as 'Uncle Jim.'[2]

Dr Rushton was also a polymath, keen on computers but also interested in DIY and working on his cars and motorhomes. He built his own car in the 1960s and converted a Ford Transit minibus into a motor caravan in which he, his wife Cynthia and their five children annually toured Europe.

The Practice at 19 Temple Close

The Huntingdon Practice that Dr Rushton joined had moved to 19 Temple Close by 1969. These premises were used until 1987 when Ermine Street surgery opened. It was a converted old people's bungalow which originally had a garden down to the river, but this had been cut in two by the new ring road. This *"tatty old bungalow"*[3] had only 2 consulting rooms, a waiting room, a room for the nurse and a kitchen (used by the staff for smoking!). Verna Hayes who used to visit with her mother, Nurse 'Mart', describes 19 Temple Place as,

> *"just a tiny bungalow and difficult to find with no parking spaces. It was an unusual place for a doctor's surgery with Peacocks Funeral Directors directly opposite!"*[4]

By 1969, the proportion of doctors in the UK working on their own had reduced to 12%,[5] and likewise the staff of the Hicks Practice was starting to grow. Nurse Eileen May started to work at Temple Close and then later moved to the surgery at Old Court Hall in 1982.[6] The Hicks Group Practice also at that time, had a branch surgery at RAF Wyton for the Forces families. A morning surgery ran with the doctors in rota and on call until the mid-1990s when the St Ives surgery took over the contract.

Dr Rushton was a considerable asset to the wider medical community, looking after the rehabilitation wards at the local hospital. He continued to provide dental anaesthetics for local practices and was also a Clinical Assistant in the 'geriatric' wards at Petersfield Hospital. Local companies also sought out and valued his occupational health advice.[7]

Other medical support in Godmanchester

By the late 1960's two more GPs, Dr France and Dr Middlemiss, had arrived in Godmanchester. They are remembered by Cynthia Green as first holding a surgery *"in a portacabin in the area next to Transart Press - now the Baptist Church."*[8] Dr France later held surgeries in the Church Hall and Dr Middlemiss established his

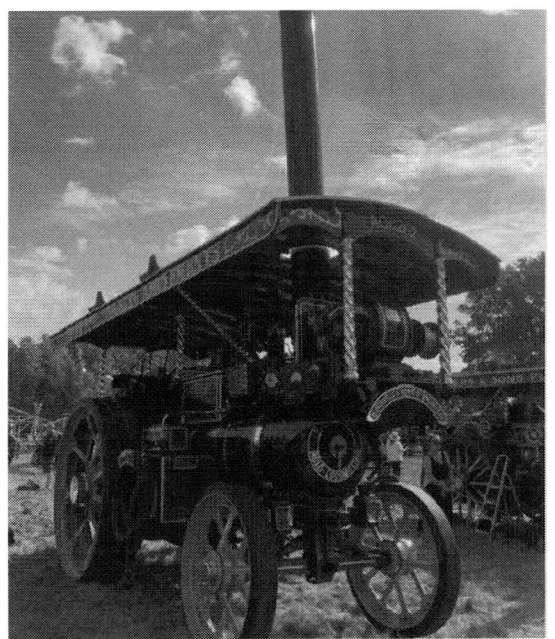
The Busy Bee today
(Courtesy of Les Williams)

surgery in Earning Street opposite the White Hart. He had his Practice there until 1985, whilst living in West Road.

Dr Middlemiss had a lifelong love of steam engines. He took five days to make the journey to Godmanchester from his native Yorkshire in his steam engine, 'The Busy Bee', which became a well-known sight around the town.[9]

Dr Middlemiss used to share a rota with the Hicks Practice doctors and Lesley Wood remembers that he was on call every 4th weekend between 6.00pm on Friday and 8.00am on Monday.[10]

MAGPAS Air Ambulance was founded in 1971 and is one of the UK's oldest emergency medical charities. It was started by two GPs from Cambridgeshire, Dr Neville Silverston and Dr Derek Cracknell. Together they recruited a network of over 100 GPs around Cambridgeshire who could be called upon day or night, to treat patients at the scene of road accidents and other emergencies, supported with the Air Ambulance if necessary.[11]

Changes at the Practice

Nelson Hicks retired from full time work at the Practice in 1973 but continued to work as a locum for the next few years. By now only 2.4% births took place at home, with 80% births in hospital. Home visits, with all the travelling and expense involved, became regarded as clinically unproductive.[12] The Hicks Group GPs began to focus on more complex chronic disease prevention as well as minor illnesses. The Practice now undertook screening for cholesterol levels, obesity, diabetes and alcohol problems.[13]

The new Labour government introduced funding for family planning services as part of general medical services in 1974, with all contraceptive advice and prescriptions free of charge on the NHS, irrespective of age or marital status.[14] More technical diagnostic equipment became available and patient expectations for 'same day appointments' increased. More staff were required due to the new demands being placed on the Practice.

Dr Keith Stewart was recruited in 1974. He joined as partner to Dr Rushton due to increased workload as Dr Hynes retired because of ill health in 1973. Keith Stewart had qualified from Guy's hospital in London and came from a medical family. His interest was in women's health and subsequently Ear, Nose and Throat (ENT) treatments. Dr Stewart left the Practice after 25 years to become an audiology consultant in Kent in 1999.[15]

Lesley Wood agrees with Keith Stewart's view of Jim Rushton's character. She says,

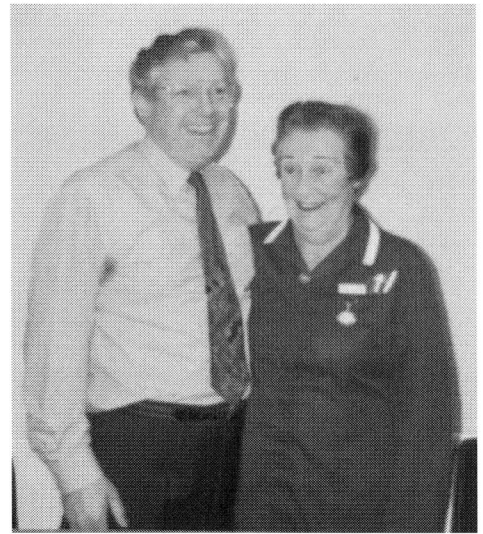

Dr Keith Stewart with Midwife Mary Moate (Charles Hicks Practice archive)

"Dr Rushton was fierce but fair. He was hopeless at remembering the names of staff and could be abrupt. But he always supported staff and once brought me a tot of Scotch whisky as a gift after he had made me upset."[16]

Dr Adelaide Turnill was the first female doctor in the Practice. She qualified from Queen's University, Belfast, and had worked as a paediatrician in Germany, where she met her husband ('Teddy' Turnill), who was the youngest colonel in the British Army at the time. He later became CEO of the Papworth Trust.

Dr Turnill joined the Practice as a part-time assistant in 1975 and became a full partner in 1976. She was hugely popular with patients, especially women and older patients. Elish Millard (now Deputy Chair of the Patients' Forum) was the Age UK manager for Huntingdonshire at the time and says, *"Dr Turnill was very helpful with all my older people, and they were very sad when she retired in 2004."*[17] Lesley Wood remembers *"…she was always dressed well and very popular with staff…but you couldn't cut corners, and everything had to be perfect."*[18]

Another major change at the Practice was introduced by Dr Rushton in 1974. An early adopter of computers himself, he was the driving force behind the Practice becoming one of the first in the area to have a computer system.

Wendy Stukins started in 1977 at Temple Close as a receptionist but soon found herself wearing other hats as new roles evolved. The photo shows Dr Rushton supervising Wendy's inputting skills on the new computer system about which he was very enthusiastic. It was used for immunisation scheduling and electronic recording of patient data for the first time.

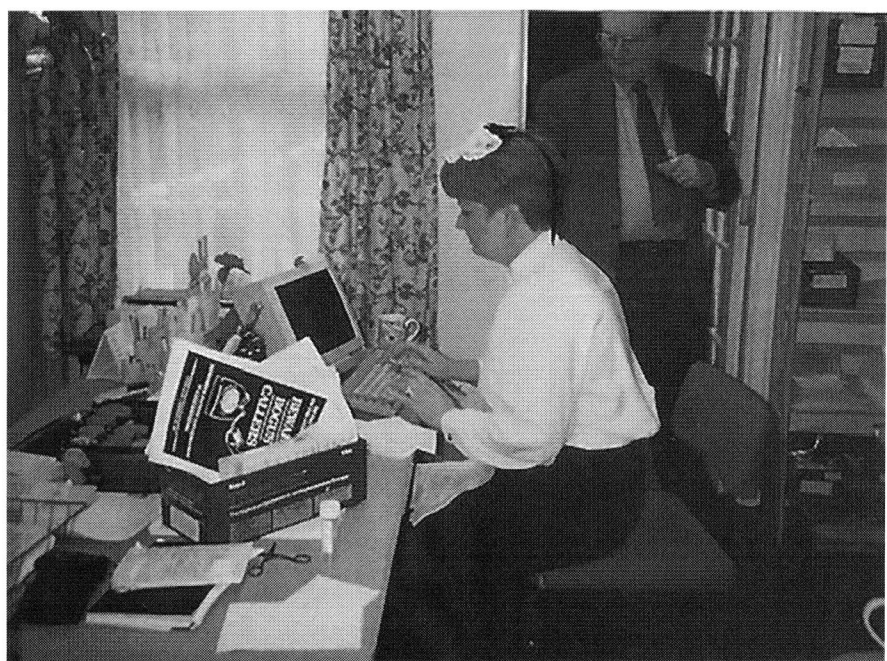

Wendy Stukins with Dr Rushton (Charles Hicks Practice archive)

A new surgery in Godmanchester

By 1983, the Practice altogether had around 8,000 patients in Huntingdon, Godmanchester and RAF Wyton.[19] The growth in population in Godmanchester to almost 3,000,[20] meant that new premises were required. It was increasingly difficult to deliver comprehensive primary care to all patients in both towns from the cramped, inadequate bungalow at Temple Close.

The new Godmanchester surgery in Old Court Hall was converted from four old, terraced houses by Dr Rushton and his 3 sons. It was a real family practice affair with everyone pitching in on the conversion.[21] Initially Old Court Hall surgery opened in 1982 as a 'branch surgery' in Godmanchester, with the ground floor having only 2 consulting rooms, 1 nurse treatment room and 1 reception area. Jim Moffat the dentist had moved his surgery from Huntingdon and had the upstairs premises – but no waiting room.

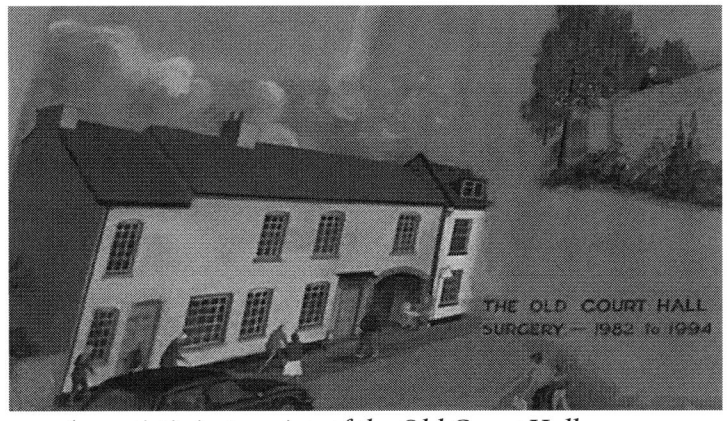

An artistic impression of the Old Court Hall surgery
(From the painting in the entrance lobby to the current Roman Gate surgery)

At first, it was difficult to offer an adequate service to patients. Wendy Stukins worked at Old Court Hall from the opening in 1982 and remembers,

"It was unfinished for months and only had one toilet. At first there was no phone, so it was 'walk in' patients only."[22]

The new computer system was slow to be installed making life difficult for new receptionist Lesley Wood.

"We had a sheet of paper on the reception desk and would write the name of each patient as they came in. Then pull their Lloyd George envelope of notes. The doctor would buzz when they were free, and we would give each patient their notes to take in. There were no appointments as it was first come, first seen. At the end of surgery, we would collect the notes from each room and file them away again. Even all those years ago, we struggled to get everyone seen."[23]

The new Hinchingbrooke Hospital opened in 1983 with 330 beds and the Maternity Hospital in Primrose Lane closed relocating to a new unit at Hinchingbrooke Hospital. In these early days of collaboration between GP practices and their local hospital, research showed that referral for specialist hospital treatment was under for 20% of patients annually. These were 4% for admission, 4% for outpatient consultation and the rest for an X-Ray or a test.[24] Mandatory vocational training for GPs had been introduced in 1982 and 'general practice now attracted its share of the best medical students.'[25]

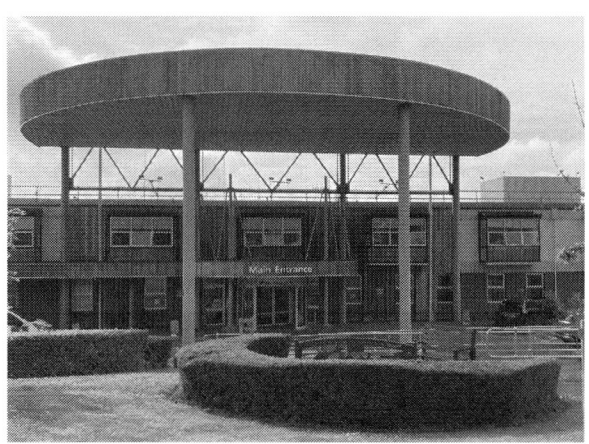

Main Hospital entrance
(Patients' Forum archive)

Dr Mike Whitton joined the team having qualified from Leeds in 1976. After starting with a GP registrar role until 1983, he was attracted to general practice being motivated by the prospect of 'continuity of care' with patients. Interested in promoting women's health, he later also focussed on occupational health.[26] He spent his whole career with the Charles Hicks Practice, retiring after 30 years, in 2013.

Dr Whitton was recruited initially to work mainly at Old Court Hall with Dr Rushton, which was just as well as Wendy Stukins recalls,

".... in his early days at Temple Close he used to make house calls on the Oxmoor Estate and often had to call us for help and directions as he was always getting

lost."[27] Doctors were only paid £20 for home visits at night and were expected to do up to 30 daytime home visits free as part of their rota.[28]

Dr Whitton remembers Jim Rushton,

"I joined the Practice in 1983 and over the years I came to know Jim well. He had a formidable intellect and had a reputation as the best diagnostician amongst us. He was considered by his peers as an excellent clinician and his second opinion was frequently sought by them. The staff trusted him implicitly, he was a skilled clinician; shrewd in business and tactful in political matters, he was a great mentor and tremendous Senior Partner."[29]

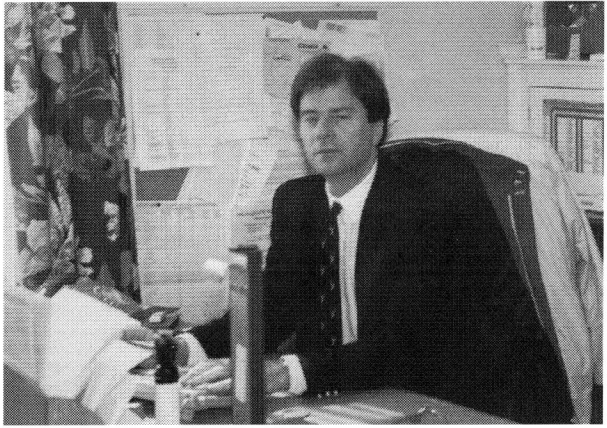

Dr Whitton at Old Court Hall
(Charles Hicks Practice archive)

Dr Whitton's appointment also heralded an increase in support staff across both surgeries. A new nurse, Irene Duckitt, was appointed, along with Sue Laxton (recruited from the District Nursing team) and Gail Evans. Sisters Jackie Baker and Jackie Parker also joined later. Valerie Cattle was head receptionist at Old Court Hall and Betty Millard was secretary. Dr Rushton did not help the induction of new staff by telling them that upstairs at Old Court Hall was haunted by the ghost of *"old Joe."*[30]

Dr Middlemiss retired in 1985 and his contribution to the doctors' rota was much missed. His Practice with mainly Godmanchester patients, was taken over by Dr Gupta, newly arrived in Godmanchester. He continued as a single doctor Practice, and his surgery was held in a bungalow in St Annes Lane (now the house of current Mayor, Alan Hooker). Dr Gupta did not join the Hicks Group doctors' rota but was well-liked by patients such as Les Williams who says *"my parents thought the world of Dr Gupta. He helped my poorly dad a lot."*[31]

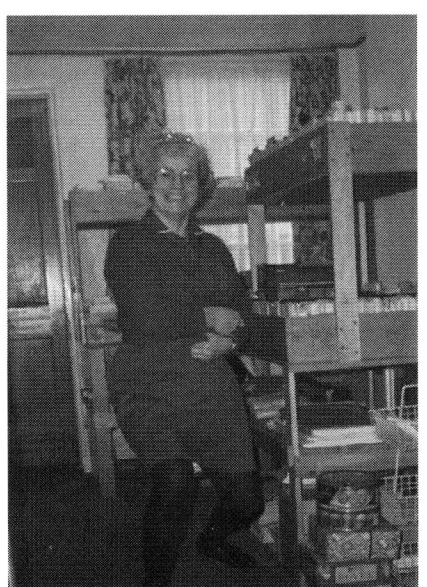

Nurse Irene Duckitt
(Charles Hicks Practice archive)

New surgeries in Huntingdon

1987 was a significant year as the Huntingdon surgery moved from Temple Close to a newly built centre in Ermine Street, which had been under construction for the previous 2 years. A new Practice Manager, Sharon Gray was appointed. She left in 1994 to be replaced by Harry Cairns.

Dr Stanger joined the Practice in 1987 having qualified at St Thomas Hospital. Another member of the medical team from a medical family, he is fondly remembered by staff as Lesley Wood recalls, *"He always wore shorts with long socks following his time in New Zealand. He was also renowned for wearing a crazy knitted hat – even when playing golf."*[32] He stayed for 27 years, not leaving until 2014. Two other long-serving staff members joined in 1989 - Jean Huff who left in 2002 and Lesley Wood who left in 2012. Discussing her long contribution to the Practice, Lesley summed up her experience as, *"Every day was different. If you could last a month, you would stay a lifetime."*[33] Another GP, Anne Lambert also joined the team at Old Court Hall in 1990.

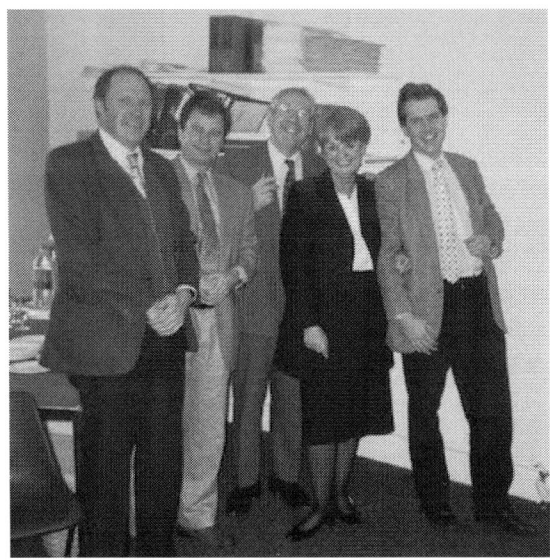
(Left to right) Dr Stanger, Dr Whitton, Dr Stewart, Wendy Stukins and Dr Sweetenham
(Charles Hicks Practice archive)

By the end of the 1980s, there were two long established medical practices in Huntingdon as Dr Connan's Practice at 84a High Street (which also had an extension flat on the growing Oxmoor Estate), moved to the current location in a new surgery next to the ring road, now known as Priory Fields. The medical team at this time were led by Dr Connan's son 'Dan', with Dr Derek Cracknell (of MAGPAS), Dr David Hunter,

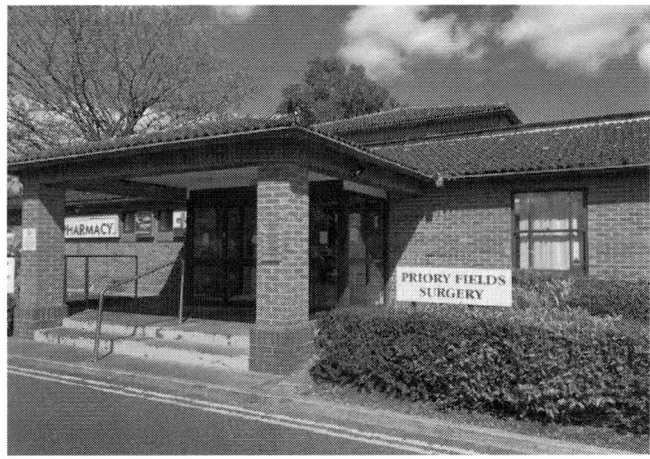
The Priory Fields Surgery on Huntingdon ring road
(Patients' Forum archive)

Dr Robert Allen, Dr Kath Lund and Dr Reynolds. Dr Rej joined in 1995 when Dan Connan retired.

The Conservative government published a White Paper – 'Promoting Better Health' in 1987. The aim was to strengthen the role of primary care in health promotion and to prevent ill health. The plan incentivised payments for GPs to increase list sizes and targeted more vaccinations, cervical screenings and health promotion.[34] This was the year of the international AIDS crisis, as well as the first successful liver, heart and lung transplant at Papworth Hospital where the patient Davina Thompson survived a further 11 years.[35]

Fund-holding rejected

In the early 1990s, another conservative government initiative was the 'Community Care Act'. This Act introduced an 'internal market model' in which GPs and health authorities could purchase services from NHS trust hospitals and other NHS providers.[36] Subsequently, district nursing, health visiting, chiropody and dietetics could also be purchased. This scheme to enable GP practices to become 'Fund Holders' and proved initially popular, with 57% English GP practices joining in. However, it was abolished within 7 years by the incoming Labour government who believed it was inefficient, expensive to operate and likely to create a 'two-tier NHS'. [37]

The Charles Hicks Practice never became a fund-holding practice being centred more on their role as advocates for patients and the community rather than financial management. As Dr Mike Whitton states, Fund-holding involved,

> *"too much administration, and the Practice partners wanted to support the new local services developing at Hinchingbrooke Hospital; unless for specialist treatment (such as neurosurgery) at Addenbrookes."*[38]

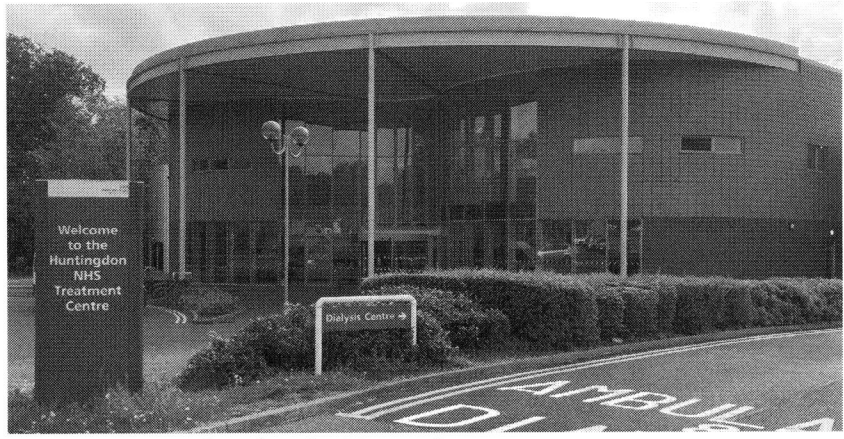

Hinchingbrooke Hospital (Patients' Forum archive)

The relationship between the Practice and Hinchingbrooke Hospital had been developing well. Dr Martin Becker was a paediatrician in the Children's Department at the Hospital between 1984 and 2011 and recalls,

"We had excellent co-operation with the Charles Hicks Practice. In addition to the usual written referrals, GPs could ring us at any time for advice or for arranging an urgent appointment, often the same day. I also found it easy to contact the GPs to discuss a particular case, or concerns about social aspects of care or neglect."[39]

Dr Becker goes on to say,

"Many GPs attended the regular Friday morning sessions at the hospital where consultants and doctors in training of all specialities came together. Invited speakers and GPs would present cases or talk on a specific topic, followed by discussions and a buffet lunch. This was particularly lively in the 80s and 90s but sadly fizzled out, presumably with GPs becoming busier and with organisational change."[40]

Developments at Ermine Street

Along with the population, patient numbers at the Huntingdon Practice continued to grow, and the Ermine Street surgery had to be extended in 1992.

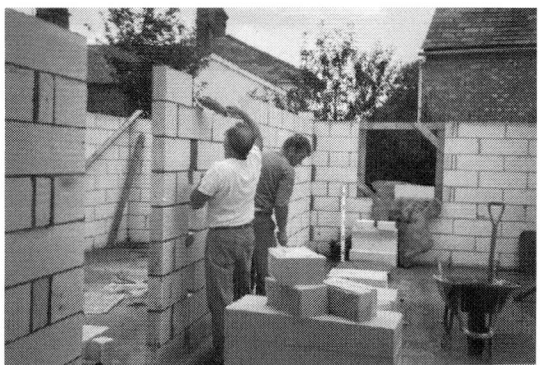
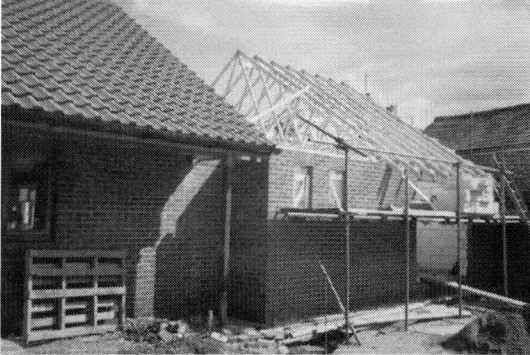

The extension underway at Ermine Street (Charles Hicks Practice archive)

Dr Sweetenham joined the Practice in 1992. He was a Cambridge graduate from a medical family following in his mother's footsteps as a GP. Like Dr Rushton he had a particular commitment at Hinchingbrooke Hospital for several years as an Ear, Nose and Throat (ENT) specialist.

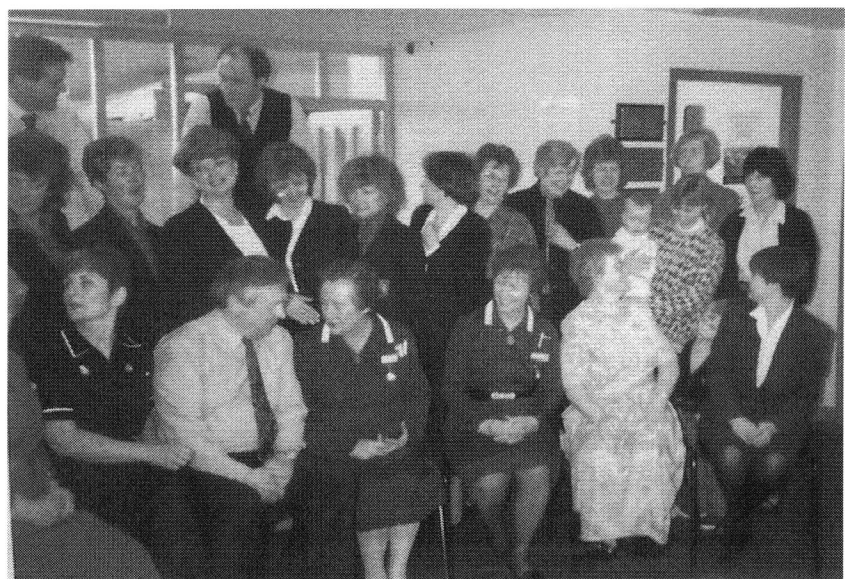

Dr Stewart and Dr Sweetenham with staff at Ermine Street
(Charles Hicks Practice archive)

Dr Rushton remained in general practice until his retirement in 1995. He and Cynthia moved to Godmanchester where they were cared for by Dr Weyell. In 2014, after the death of his wife Cynthia, he moved to Hampshire, to live with his daughter. Having survived several bouts of illness he was nicknamed 'Lazarus' by his family until his death in 2021.

Dr Sweetenham's eulogy remembers his mentor as follows:

"Jim Rushton's last few years working in general practice overlapped with my first few. He was very much the senior partner and would give wise counsel but usually in very few words. His remarks would end up describing me as 'boy'. His dedication to his Practice and patients has been displayed in the hundreds of comments received from former patients on the various social media sites. He was considered an excellent clinician by his peers as and his second opinion was frequently sought. We hope he would be proud that the Huntingdon GP COVID vaccination centre at Ermine Street is the surgery he created and worked in. The very first vaccination was given in Jim's room."[41]

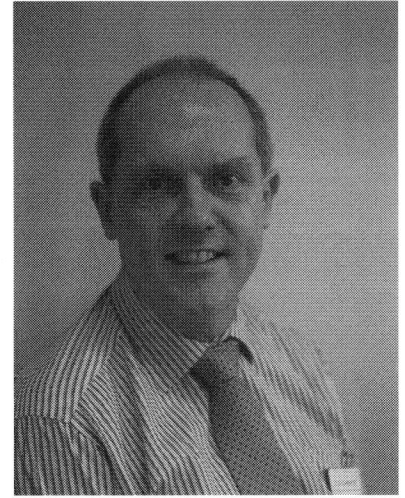

Dr I Sweetenham
(Charles Hicks Practice archive)

A final note on 'Transactions'

Dr Rushton was given 'Transactions of the Huntingdonshire Medical Society' when Nelson Hicks retired in 1973. He later donated it to the Huntingdon Library Archives where it can be found today. He also donated a collection of 19th Century medical instruments from Dr Michael Foster to the Norris Museum in St Ives, and these are featured in Chapter 3 of this book. Chapter 8 brings us up to the present day.

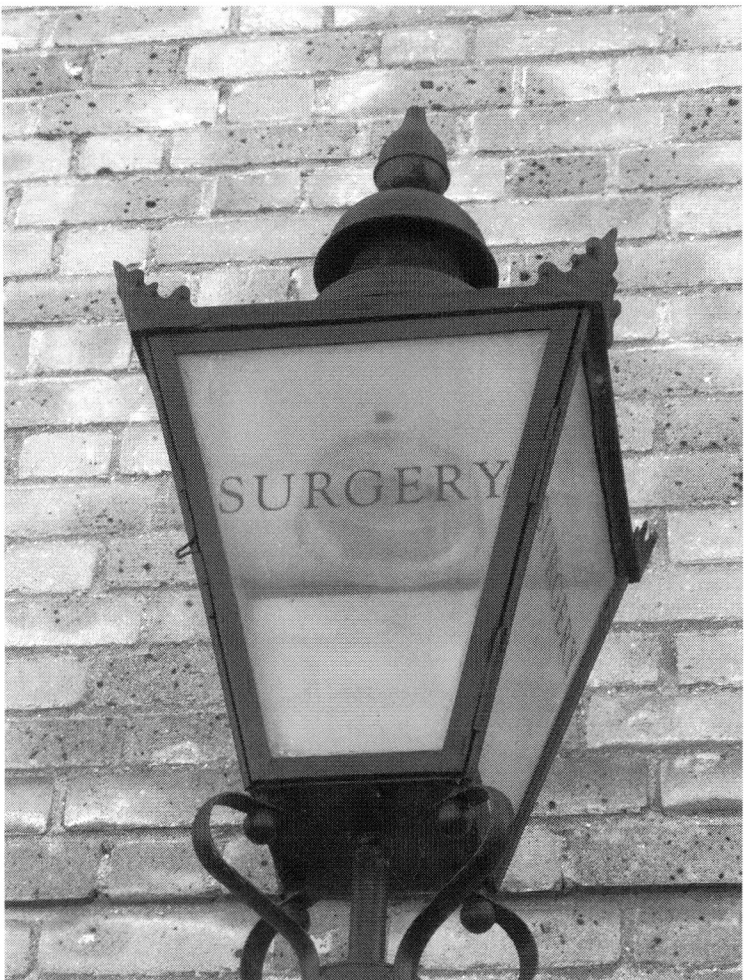

Surgery lamp
(Patients' Forum archive)

Chapter 8

The Hicks Group Practice (1994–2024) Up to the present day

The Roman Gate surgery in Godmanchester

From 1990 onwards, the development of new housing estates in Godmanchester brought a further influx of patients. The Hicks Group Practice purchased land for new surgery to be built on the site of Jack Trigwell's garage. The surgery was expanded and relocated to Pinfold Lane in March 1994 as the Roman Gate Surgery. The architect was Colin Lambert, the husband of Dr Anne Lambert who worked at Old Court Hall until 1993. The builders, David Jarvis Construction of Newmarket, had constructed the Ermine Street surgery. The new surgery was opened by Tom Dighton, one of the oldest lifelong Godmanchester residents and a patient at the Surgery.

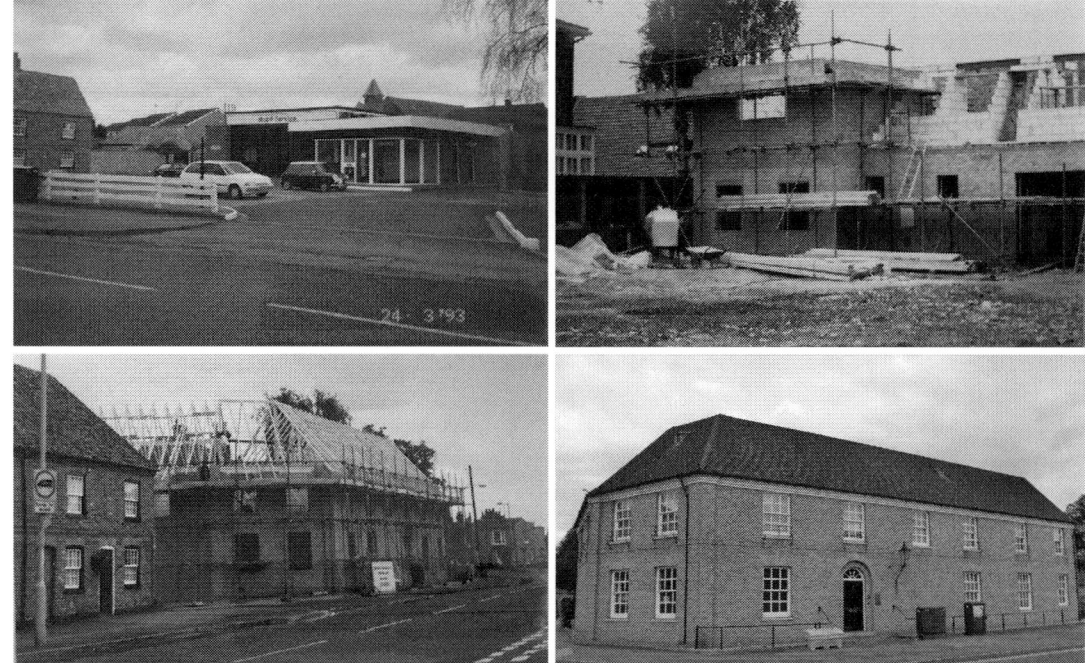

The new Roman Gate surgery under construction in 1993 (Charles Hicks Practice archive)

Expanded premises gave the opportunity for new recruitment of medical staff. Dr Richard Weyell joined the Practice in 1993 and Dr Harriet Platten became the second female GP at the Practice, when she joined in 1994. Dr Weyell had trained at the London Hospital. He was interested in the treatment of drug and alcohol abuse and became computer lead for the Practice when Dr Rushton retired. From 1997, Dr Weyell was instrumental in negotiating the Personal Medical Services (PMS) contracts with the relevant NHS funding providers, eventually retiring through ill health in 2020. Dr Platten was a rheumatology specialist who qualified at Bristol University and retired in 2008.[1]

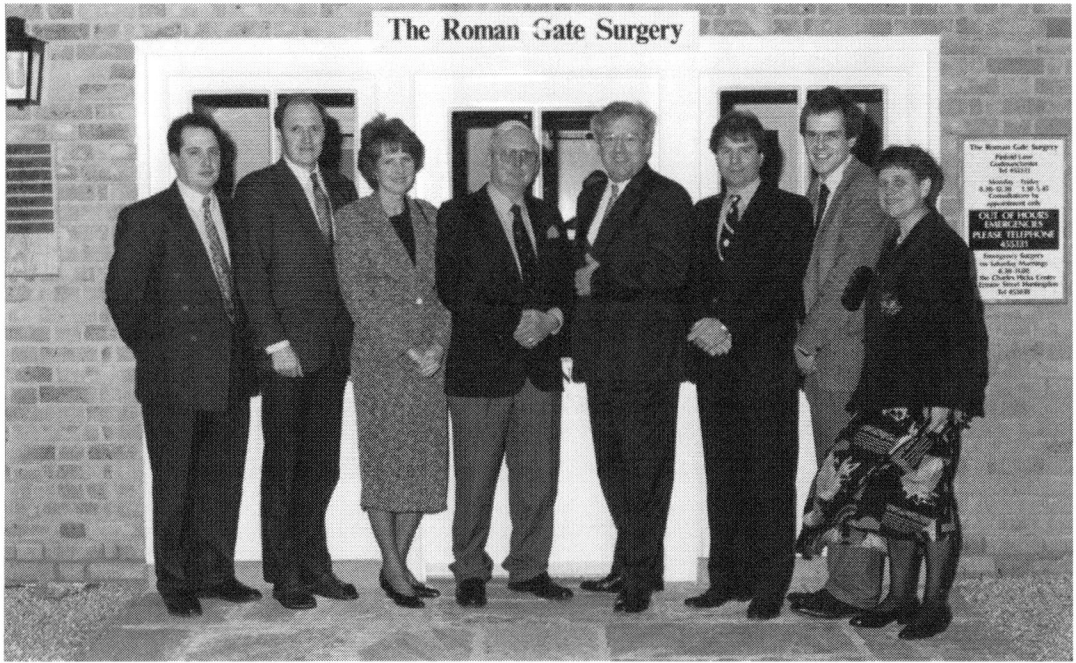

The opening of the Roman Gate surgery in 1994 with (left to right) Dr Richard Weyell, Dr John Stanger, Dr Adelaide Turnill, Dr Jim Rushton, Dr Keith Stewart, Dr Michael Whitton, Dr Ian Sweetenham, Dr Harriet Platten. (Charles Hicks Practice archive)

With the new premises came significant changes, although not all at once. Nationally, by 1995, around 90% of GP practices had been computerised.[2] The Hicks Practice was now using their upgraded IT system for scheduling appointments as well as managing prescriptions and other administration. However, clinical notes were

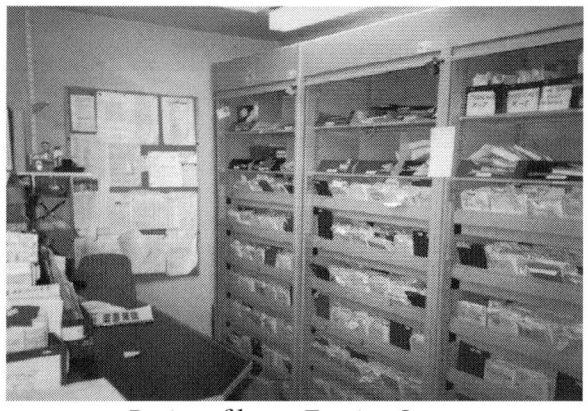

Patient files at Ermine Street
(Charles Hicks Practice archive)

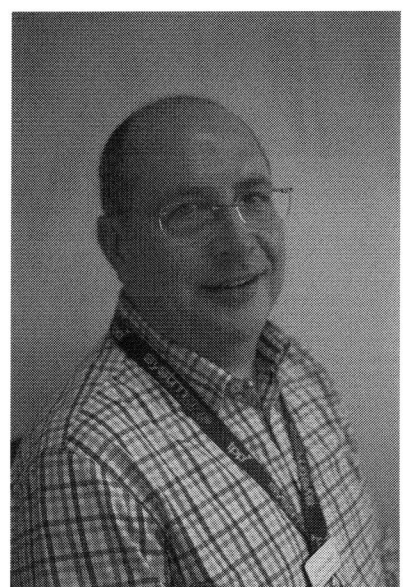

Dr R Weyell
(Charles Hicks Practice archive)

still made on paper. Lesley Wood remembers that at Ermine Street, "We were still filing patient notes in Lloyd George envelopes"[3] and Wendy Stukins says, *"I was promoted from receptionist to prescription clerk but often couldn't read the doctor's hand-writing!"*[4]

New clinics and services

GPs had agreed a new contract for the 1990s which gave financial incentives for immunisation, screening services and health promotion. This led to the recruitment nationally of many more practice nurses.[5] Asthma clinics led by nurses and antenatal clinics led by midwives began in both the Roman Gate and Ermine Street surgeries. Other clinics for child health, diabetes, rheumatology and dermatology were led by the doctors.[6]

By 1995, 78% of people were consulting their GP at least once a year.[7] The population was becoming increasingly accustomed to consumerism and 24-hour services and wanted primary health care to be available on the same basis.[8] In 1996 'Hunts Doc' formed to enable practices to share the out of hours rota.[9]

The year 1997 saw the election of a new Labour government and significant changes began. Alan Milburn, one of the first Health Secretaries under Tony Blair, stated that: *"The NHS is a 1940s system operating in a 21st century world."*[10] Fund holding practices established under the Thatcher government were abolished.

A new NHS (Primary Care) Act enabled health authorities to commission a new style Personal Medical Services (PMS) contract with local primary care practices for a defined package of services. This contract enabled salaried doctors to be employed by practices. In 1999, income from working with Addenbrooke's Hospital to provide training for medical students appears in the Hicks Practice accounts for the first time and continues today.

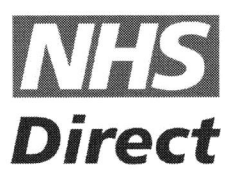

The famous 'blue lozenge' logo for NHS services began to feature on both NHS and new privatised initiatives.[11] NHS Direct was launched nationally in 1998 as a telephone triage service staffed by nurses. In the same year, Care UK began to open Care Direct walk-in centres in cities for those who could not access GP services at hours to suit them.[12]

Changes in Huntingdon and Godmanchester

Changes in medical provision were underway in Godmanchester and Huntingdon. The Acorn Surgery opened in March 2001 on the Oxmoor Estate, having initially been based in temporary accommodation on the site of Huntingdon College, whilst the Oak Tree Centre was being built. During the first two years this Practice became the fastest growing GP Practice in the history of the NHS![13]

Priory Fields had no further capacity and closed their list at this time. Two of the 'Acorn doctors' – Dr Boyle and Dr Stanton ran extra surgeries at Ermine Street until the Acorn Centre was fully open.[14]

In 2002 Dr Gupta retired and closed his Practice in Godmanchester. His patients moved either to Roman Gate or one of the rapidly expanding Huntingdon surgeries.[15]

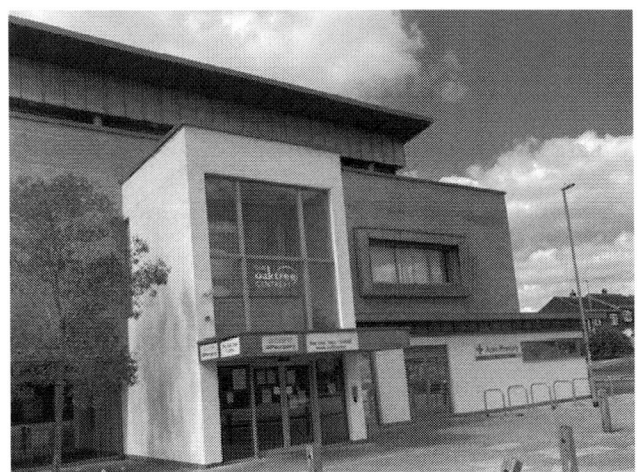

The Acorn Surgery at the Oak Tree Centre in Huntingdon (Patients' Forum archive)

The first salaried doctor was employed by the Hicks Practice under the PMS contract. He was Dr Heinz van Raemdonck, recruited to help the Roman Gate surgery cope with increase in patient numbers moving across from Dr Gupta's Practice in Godmanchester.

A new GP contract was agreed in 2004 with 79% of GPs nationally backing the deal. The contract offered a pay rise to GPs with the average income rising from £65,000 to £80,000 per year. There was also an end to evening and weekend working with local Primary Care Trusts contracted to provide cover as out of hours care became financially unsustainable under the new contract.[16] Although welcomed by some GPs (and their families), the loss of 24-hour responsibility for patients inevitably meant some diminution of patient contact.[17]

At the same time 'performance-related payment' was introduced through the Quality Outcomes Framework (QOF).[18] Practices were set new targets for evidence of chronic disease management such as heart disease and diabetes. Data was also recorded for providing appointments within 48 hours, improved patient satisfaction and narrowing health inequalities whilst reaching benchmark costs of care.[19]

Dr Stanger and Dr Sweetenham were QOF assessors who helped establish the QOF process locally. The launch of the NHS Choices website was intended to give

The Hicks Group Practice (1994–2024)

patients accurate and up to date health information and enabled them to monitor the performance of their practice.[20]

In 2006, Dr Sweetenham established an Ear, Nose and Throat (ENT) clinic for the Huntingdon area at the Roman Gate surgery. Dr Smithson joined the Hicks Practice in the same year and remains as a partner in 2024. She qualified from Sheffield in 1998 and specialises in gynaecology, contraception, paediatrics and minor surgery as well as supervising trainee doctors at the Practice.

Dr Tolliss also joined the Practice in 2006 and left in 2020, returning later as a locum GP.

Dr Soni joined the Practice in 2011 and today remains as a partner with lead responsibility for trainee doctors. He also has special interests in diabetes, dermatology, ophthalmology and minor surgery.

Dr Sophie Densem also joined at this time and remains as a salaried GP today.

2012 Health and Social Care Act

The Health and Social Care Act introduced by the coalition government '*heralded the most far - ranging reforms of the NHS since its launch in 1948.*'[21] The Act created an internal market in health care with Clinical Commissioning Groups (CCGs) replacing Primary Care Trusts (PCTs) with responsibility for contracting most health services, including GP practices. The Care Quality Commission (CQC) began a programme of inspections of GP surgeries in 2013.[22]

Growing local populations continued to increase demands on both the Roman Gate and Ermine Street surgeries. By 2011 the Godmanchester population had increased in 10 years by over 700 residents (12%) and the Huntingdon population by 3,600 (18%). Rising workloads for the surgery staff

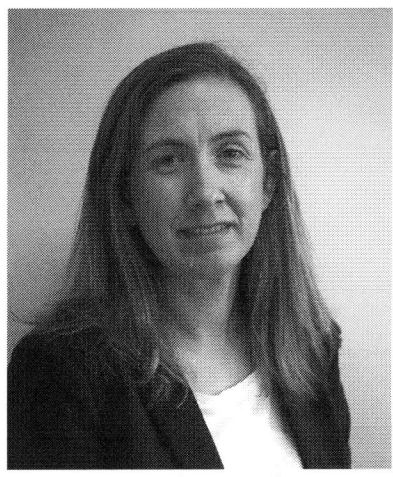

Dr Carolyn Smithson
(Charles Hicks Practice archive)

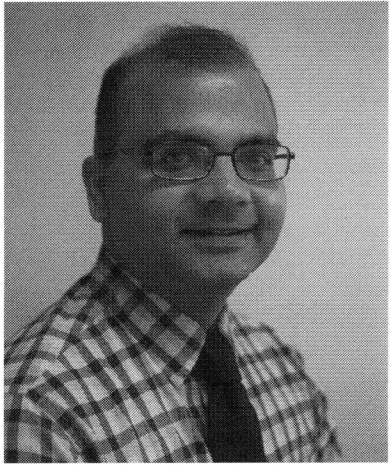

Dr Urjit Soni
(Charles Hicks Practice archive)

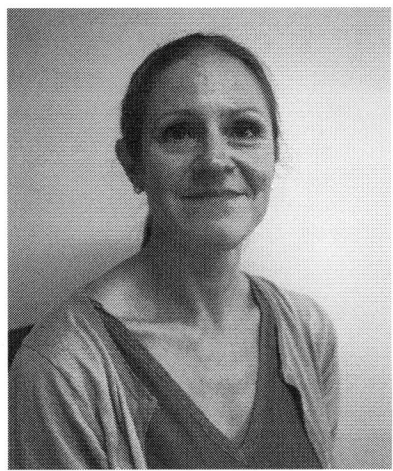

Dr Sophie Densem
(Charles Hicks Practice archive)

also resulted from an increase in the number of consultations per patient. Nationally the average patient consulted their GP practice 6.7 times per year, compared to 3.9 times in 1995. The biggest increase was among patients aged over 70 as the impact of an ageing population with multiple conditions became apparent.[23]

The Patients' Forum

In 2009 the forerunner of the Patients' Forum was set up. It was among the first 'Patient Participation Groups' (PPGs) in Cambridgeshire. The Group was actively supported by Dr Whitton, who recruited Sandy Ferrelly, a local Godmanchester resident as Chair. Sandy had recently retired as a senior administrator at St Thomas Hospital in London and knew the working of the NHS well. Sandy was Chair of the Group, re-named as the Patients' Forum for almost 10 years before retiring due to ill health. Sandy died peacefully at home in January 2024.

Other original committee members who have made great contributions to the Patients' Forum over the years include Merle Bailey, Maggie Middlemiss, John Thackray, Martyn and Pat Fox and Elish Millard (who remains vice-chair 12 years later).

Increasing patient expectations of levels of service made the role of the Patients' Forum very timely, helping to improve communication to and from the Practice.

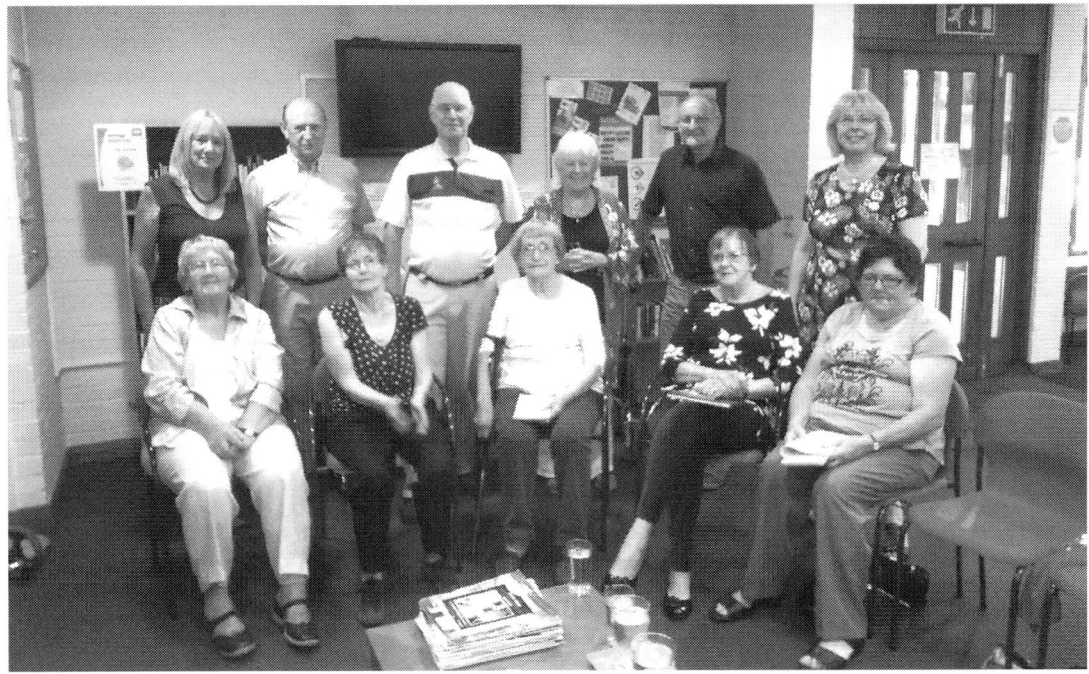

Patients Group photo from 2015 with back row (left to right): Maggie Middlemiss, John Thackray, Martyn Fox, Elish Millard, Roger Merritt, Janice Ballard. Front row: Anne James, Pat Fox, Pat Wilson, Sandy Ferrelly, and Pat Jones.

(Patients' Forum archive)

The Forum aims to provide a voice for all Hicks Group patients in Godmanchester and Huntingdon, providing feedback on patient services to the Practice staff and working with other organisations to inform patients about sources of further support. They also raise funds for equipment and improved Practice facilities. The Forum team publish regular newsletters and meet patients to gather feedback and explain the introduction of new ways to access treatment at the Practice such as the NHS App, telephone triage and online consultations.

Support staff continue to increase

The role of new support staff became increasingly important with the opportunity for Nursing Practitioners and Healthcare Assistants to work alongside the GPs.[24] Zoe Dickson was the first at the Hicks Practice to be trained as a Nurse Practitioner and be able to prescribe.[25] She gained her Bachelor of Science (First Class Honours) as Advanced Nurse Practitioner in July 2005 and her Certificate in Non-Medical Prescribing in April 2007.

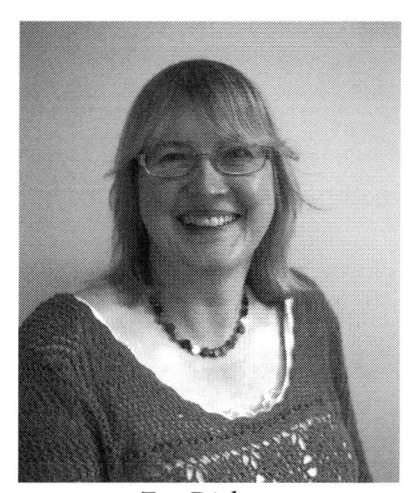

Zoe Dickson
(Charles Hicks Practice archive)

By 2014, female GPs outnumbered male GPs in England for the first time.[26] At the Hicks Group Practice, staff numbers continued to increase as a Multidisciplinary Team began to be created. There were 7 GPs (5 males and 2 females) plus 2 trainee Doctors (both females). The Practice nursing team of 8, was made up of 1 Nurse Practitioner (Zoe Dickson), a Lead Nurse (Karen Moseley) with 5 Practice Nurses and a Healthcare Assistant. Also, a Practice Manager (Lorraine Baker) and an Assistant Practice Manager (Lisa Harrison – now Practice Manager 10 years later). The administration team of 9 had 2 Medical Secretaries, a Prescription Clerk and 6 Administrator/Receptionists. This was also the year that NHS Direct was replaced by NHS 111.

For many practices, the continuity of personal care became more challenging to maintain: *"Continuity as traditionally understood is becoming a thing of the past."*[27] However, the Hicks Group Practice had a CQC inspection report in 2016 which rated the Practice as 'Good' with both QOF data and the National GP survey showing that patients rated the Practice higher than average for most aspects of care although 'it could be difficult to obtain routine appointments with the clinician of choice.'[28]

Coping with COVID and its impact

By 2020 a further extension had been added at the Roman Gate surgery to cope with the increased number of patients from the Romans Edge housing development in Godmanchester.

In March of 2020, the first cases of the COVID pandemic had been recognised. Dr Sweetenham recalls,

> "At the Hicks Group we had no supplies of masks and premises that were not designed for ventilation or reducing the risk of passing respiratory viruses. The surgery rapidly moved to a phone consultation model with changes in IT so that we could communicate with patients via text and be sent pictures from patients."[29]

When Huntingdon needed a Covid vaccination site the Charles Hicks Centre in Ermine Street was used. An extra door was created into the car park. All the other medical care for Hicks Group patients was delivered from the Roman Gate Surgery. The vaccinations were administered by staff from the Hicks Group, Priory Fields, Acorn and Papworth surgeries with assistance from many volunteers. Dr Stanger came out of retirement and did vaccination sessions. Irena Hall recalls the emotions of the first vaccination sessions,

> "The most elderly patients were the first to be vaccinated and they were so grateful to the staff who were risking their own health to help. We were given chocolates and other gifts and listened to many personal reminiscences from those waiting their turn for the first Pfizer vaccines."[30]

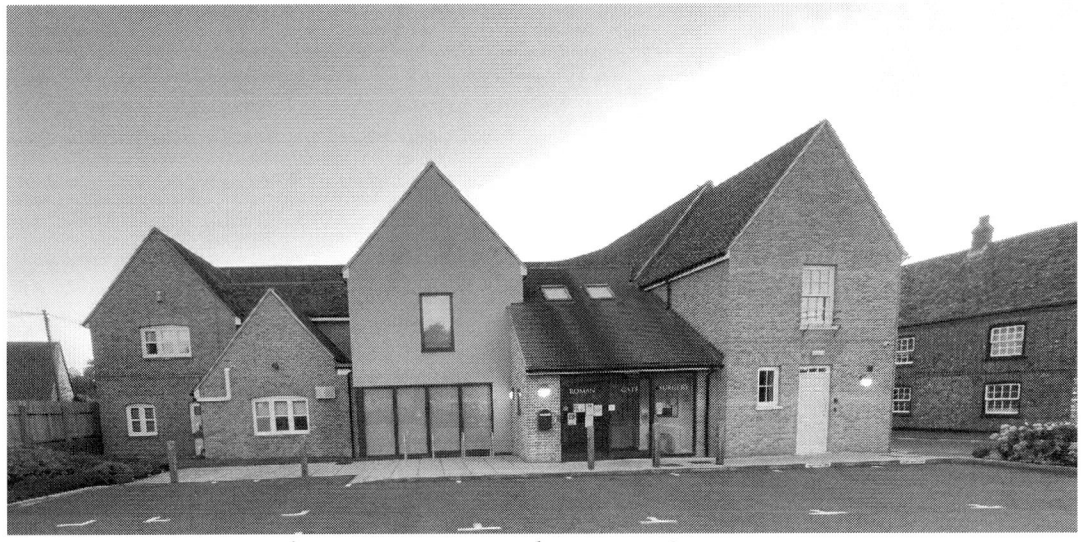

The new extension at the Roman Gate surgery
(Patients' Forum archive)

Up to the present day

By the census of 2021 the population of Godmanchester had increased by 17% in the last 10 years to just under 8,000. Huntingdon had grown at a slightly slower rate of 7% to 25,500.

Dr Bulstrode joined as a partner in 2020 plus the salaried GPs Dr Venkat Raman and Dr Grady in 2022 and in 2023, Dr Olufemi, Dr Jamie Jackson and Dr Wu. In 2024, Dr Venkat-Raman and Dr Wu became partners, so the Practice currently has 6 doctors as Partners, 4 salaried GPs plus 2 locum GPs and 7 trainee doctors taking the Practice up to its' full complement.

However, GP workload continues to be extreme with the national average number of patients per GP (Nov 2023) at 2,290 (up 6.9% since 2019), and GP staff delivering 340 million appointments in 2022 (up 9% more than in 2019).[31] The total number of patients registered with the Hicks Group Practice is currently almost 17,000.

More 'top down' NHS reorganisation was introduced in the Health and Care Act of 2022. This Act was intended to make it easier for health and care organisations to deliver 'joined up care' for patients who rely on multiple services from NHS organisations, local authorities, the voluntary and community sector and other providers.[32]

For Primary Care, the Local Integrated Care Boards (ICBs) fund GP practices and Primary Care Networks (PCNs) to work with an Additional Roles Reimbursement Scheme (ARRS). ARRS offers shared extended services throughout the Hicks Group and other local Primary Care practices. These ARRS services currently include Care Co-ordinators, Clinical Pharmacists, a Community Matron, Health and Wellbeing Coaches, Dementia Support workers and Social Prescribers. Together with Practice staff, this forms a full 'Multi-disciplinary Team'. However staffing and resourcing challenges continue to increase, with only £14.9 billion (8%) of the total £190 billion of the NHS budget currently spent on Primary Care and an ongoing dispute over the 2024/25 contract with NHS England (NHSE).[33]

A national and local view of the future

GP workload remains a key issue and nationally GP numbers (Nov 2023) were 27,482 full time equivalent (FTE) GPs – 2.3% less than December 2019 (and 6.4% less than in 2015).[34] Around 68% GPs nationally say they don't have enough time to adequately assess and treat patients or build the patient relationships needed to deliver quality care. GPs also work on average 10 hours more than their contracted hours each week and 42% say they are planning to quit the profession in the next 5 years.[35]

From a local staff perspective, there is no doubt that the pressure of workload at the Hicks Group Practice continues to increase. The volume of calls from patients seeking appointments at times seems unmanageable in reception, even now with the addition of a popular 'call back' telephone system. The NHS App does enable new messaging systems, although some elderly patients find smartphone technology difficult or unaffordable. Other patients can appear to have unrealistic expectations but may not appreciate constraints on human resources and budgets at the Practice.[36]

Many challenges for the NHS continue in 2024 and beyond. Hospital doctors of all grades, along with nurses and other healthcare professionals have been, and some continue to be, involved in industrial action about contracts and pay. This has impacted on Primary Care, with some of the trainee doctors striking. Long waiting lists for hospital treatment mean that some patients increasingly need more support than ever from their GP and clinical support team.

One of the Practice partners, Dr Carolyn Smithson concludes

"Our Hicks Group Practice prides itself on offering an outstanding level of service to our nearly 17,000 patients. Our feedback is overwhelmingly positive, with patients appreciative of the friendly team and excellent clinical care. We continue to be at the forefront of innovation, whilst maintaining a responsive, caring service for our patients. The future will no doubt throw further challenges at us, but we are ready to face them."[37]

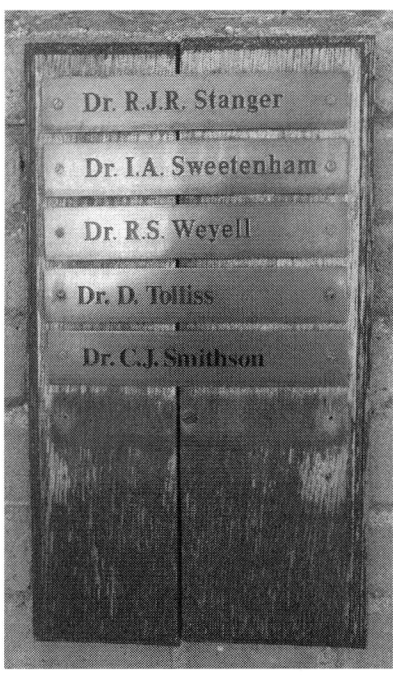

Appendix 1

Timeline for the Charles Hicks Practice

Huntingdonshire Medical Society (1793– 1803)
1789	Dispensary in Huntingdon established
1798	Vaccination by cowpox to prevent smallpox began by Edward Jenner
1799	Seven Huntingdon parishes subscribe to access Addenbrooke's Hospital, Cambridge
1804	Workhouse opened in Huntingdon

Jonah Wilson (1809–1848)
1815	Apothecaries Act
1816	Stethoscope invented by Rene Laennec in France
1817	Smallpox vaccinations in Godmanchester administered by Robert Fox
1823	The Lancet founded by Thomas Wakley
1828	New prison opened in Huntingdon
1831	Infirmary added to Huntingdon dispensary
1831/32	First cholera outbreak
1832	Anatomy Act
1834	Poor Law Amendment Act
1837	New workhouse opened in Huntingdon
1842	Edwin Chadwick's report into sanitary conditions and public health
1844	Ether used in dentistry by Horace Wells in USA

Michael Foster (1833–1876)
1846	First operation under anaesthesia by Robert Liston
1847	James Simpson discovered the use of chloroform as an anaesthetic
1847	Ignaz Semmelweis introduced hand washing into gynaecology
1848	First Public Health Act
1848/49	Second cholera outbreak
1849	John Snow's report on mode of communication of cholera in London
1853	Huntingdon Town and County hospital founded
1853	Smallpox vaccination Act

1853/4 First hypodermic needle invented by Alexander Wood in Scotland
1855   British Medical Association founded
1858   The Medical Register and the General Medical Council founded
1860   Florence Nightingale's Nursing School founded at St Thomas Hospital
1860   The Three Counties Hospital opened in Bedfordshire
1862   First paid female health visitors appointed in Manchester
1864   Germ theory expounded by Louis Pasteur
1865   Experiments with antiseptic treatment began by Joseph Lister
1866   First clinical thermometer developed by Thomas Allbutt

Herbert Lucas (1863–1919)
1872   Carbolic spray introduced by Joseph Lister
1875   Second Public Health Act
1881   Tuberculosis bacillus identified by Robert Koch
1890   Thomas Halstead in USA began wearing surgical gloves
1895   X rays discovered by Wilhelm Roentgen in Germany
1898   Huntingdon Infectious Disease hospital opened
1902   Radium discovered by Pierre and Marie Curie
1902   Midwives Act (established the Central Midwives Board)
1903   Bosworth House surgery opened in Huntingdon
1907   Salversan 606 discovered to treat syphilis

Charles Hicks (1910–1948)
1909   First state pension introduced for men and women over 70
1910   The workhouse became Walnut Tree House
1911   National Insurance Act
1914   Walden House Voluntary Aid hospital opened for wounded servicemen
1919   Nurses' Registration Act
1928   Experiments with penicillin began by Alexander Fleming
1929   Papworth village settlement for TB patients established
1936   Midwives Act (gave Local Authorities responsibility for midwife services)
1939   Experiments with penicillin continued by Howard Florey
1939   Paxton Park maternity hospital opened
1942   Beveridge report
1948   National Health Service began
1948   Walnut Tree House joined the NHS as Petersfield Hospital

Hicks Practice timeline and partners to the present day

Nelson Hicks (1948–1973)
1950	Collings Report on GP practice standards
1960	Primrose Lane maternity hospital opened
1965	Family Doctor Charter
1969	The Hicks Practice moved to 19 Temple Close
1970	Area Health Authorities established
1971	MAGPAS Air ambulance founded

Jim Rushton (1965–1995)
1974	Dr Keith Stewart (to 1999)
1975	Dr Adelaide Turnill (to 2004)
1982	Godmanchester surgery opened in Old Court Hall
1982	Branch surgery at RAF Wyton (to 1995)
1983	Medical Act established specialist general managers
1983	Hinchingbrooke Hospital opened with 330 beds
1983	Primrose Lane maternity hospital closed and relocated to Hinchingbrooke Hospital
1983	Dr Mike Whitton (to 2013)
1985	AIDS epidemic
1987	New surgery opened at Ermine Street, Huntingdon
1987	Promoting Better Health report incentivised GP payments
1987	Dr John Stanger (to 2014)
1989	Fund holding started giving GPs control over budgets
1989	Priory Fields practice opened in present location
1990	Community Care Act established new NHS Trusts
1992	Ermine Street surgery extended
1992	Dr Ian Sweetenham (to present)
1993	Dr Richard Weyell (to 2020)
1994	New Roman Gate surgery opened in Godmanchester
1994	Dr Harriet Platten (to 2008)

Hicks Group practice (1995 –2024)
1997	Fund holding ended
1997	Primary Care Act
2001	Acorn surgery opened in Huntingdon
2004	QOF introduced with evidence based targets for GPs
2006	Dr Carolyn Smithson (to present)

2006	Dr Tollis (to 2020)
2009	Patients' Forum founded
2011	Dr Urjit Soni (to present)
2011	Dr Sophie Densem (to present)
2012	Health and Social Care Act established Clinical Commissioning Groups (CCGs)
2013	CQC inspections began
2020	Extension added to Roman Gate surgery
2020	COVID pandemic
2020	Dr Sean Bulstrode (to present)
2020	Dr Venkat Raman (to present)
2022	Health and Care Act established Integrated Care Boards (ICBs) and Primary Care Networks (PCNs)
2023	Dr Wu (to present)

(With grateful thanks to Dr Mike Muncaster for the origins of this Timeline)

Appendix 2

Women and Healthcare

The first woman doctor appointed in the Charles Hicks Practice was Adelaide Turnill in 1975. There were many other women who have played a role in treating sickness in the community over the 200 years of our story. Some of their names we know but most remain hidden. This Appendix pays tribute to them all.

The herbalists

Largely excluded from the history of formal medical practice, are local women with medical knowledge and experience shared and passed on for centuries. As carers and mothers in the 19th century, many women possessed skills and knowledge that should not be overlooked. They delivered tonics and herbal remedies to families and the community as required. Many early apothecaries such as Jonah Wilson gained prestige from writing about and often selling, these same herbs and preparations as proprietary medicines.[1]

The midwives

Traditionally considered a woman's role, men were not allowed into the birthing room. By the beginning of the 19th century, the man-midwife began to be used by those who could afford to pay for a physician or surgeon to attend a birth. Local women remained important for other birthing rituals and as a source of support during and after home births up to the mid-20th century.[2] We have seen the importance of long-serving District Nurses such as Doreen Mart, Nurse Moate and Nurse Meeks from the 1950s onwards. At the Practice now, there are also female Community Midwives and Health Visitors.

Hospital Matrons

Links between GPs and the local hospital remain strong. At the County Hospital, Miss Armitage was appointed Matron in 1912, training and managing Red Cross nurses at Walden House, supervised by Charles Hicks during WW1. She retired in 1936, but due to the acute staffing

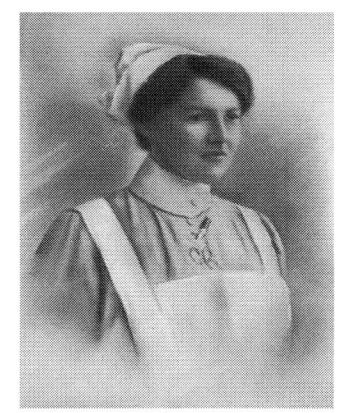

WWI Red Cross nurse
(Charles hicks Practice archive)

crisis during WW2, she was persuaded to return as Matron. With no domestic staff available, she often cooked the meals for patients and staff, as well as undertaking all her duties as Matron. She recruited all nursing and domestic staff – many of whom she had previously trained. She finally retired in 1954 after 42 years of service.[3]

The Nurses and Healthcare assistants

The first professional register of nurses was in 1919, state enrolled nurse training began in 1940, and the role of nurses in GP practices was prioritised under the NHS. The professionalisation of nurse training and recruitment of healthcare assistant continues. At the current Charles Hicks Practice there are 3 Advanced Nurse Practitioners, 5 General Nurses (of which 4 are Specialist Nurses) and 3 Healthcare Assistants. All are female.

Early doctors

Gaining access to qualifications as a medical practitioner continued to be a long battle for women throughout the 19th century. It was not until 1908 that Royal Colleges of Surgeons and Physicians admitted women to gain qualifications on the same terms as men.[4] Once qualified, becoming employed in a hospital remained a challenge and many women doctors worked overseas or moved into general practice. An unnamed qualified 'lady doctor' applied for the vacant post of House Surgeon at the County Hospital in 1911 but was not accepted.[5] In 1911, there were less than 500 registered women doctors in England and Wales, [6] compared to 2024 when now 18,900 female doctors make up 56% of the total GPs in general practice in the UK.[7]

20th century doctors

Dr Anne Connan was the first qualified woman doctor in Huntingdon, working at the Priory Fields Practice from WW2 onwards. Having qualified in 1923, Anne worked for the Malaysia Medical Service, returning to Huntingdon to support Dr Peter Connan. She was a Deputy Medical office of Health and Assistant School Medical Officer. Dr Kath Lund was the next woman doctor appointed at Priory Fields in the 1980s.

At the Charles Hicks Practice, Dr Harriet Platten was appointed in 1994, followed by Dr Carolyn Smithson in 2006 and Dr Sophie Densem in 2011, both of whom are still in post today. Women GPs

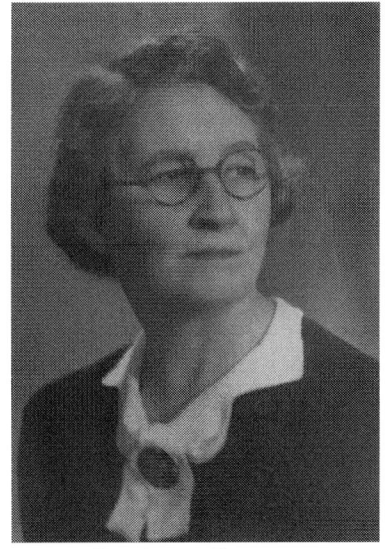

Dr. Anne Connan
(Courtesy of Dr Alex Connan)

outnumbered men nationally by 2014,[8] and at the Practice today there are 4 female and 6 male permanent GPs. The Practice has almost as many women patients as men, and the opportunity to choose to see a female doctor is often welcomed.

Other Practice staff

The Practice Manager is a key role in any practice that is often overlooked, in the last 30 years the Charles Hicks Practice has had three exceptionally talented and hard - working women managers – Sharon Grey, Lorraine Baker and Lisa Harrison.

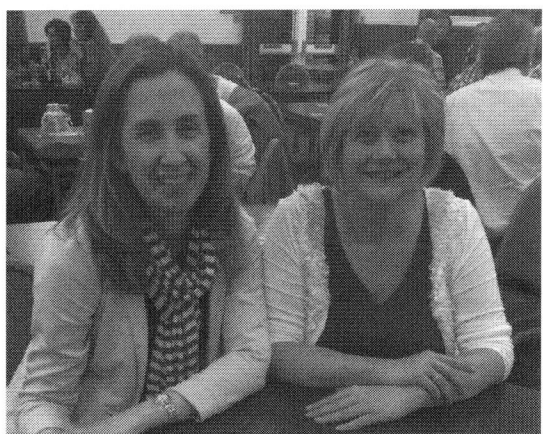

Dr Smithson and Lorraine Baker
(Patients' forum archive)

Receptionists are sometimes now referred to as 'care navigators' and the team of 12 women at the Practice are usually the first point of contact for over 16,000 patients. They play a key role in prioritising and scheduling appointments with the most suitable practitioner. The Practice is also supported with a team of 19 administrative and secretarial staff, only one of whom is male.

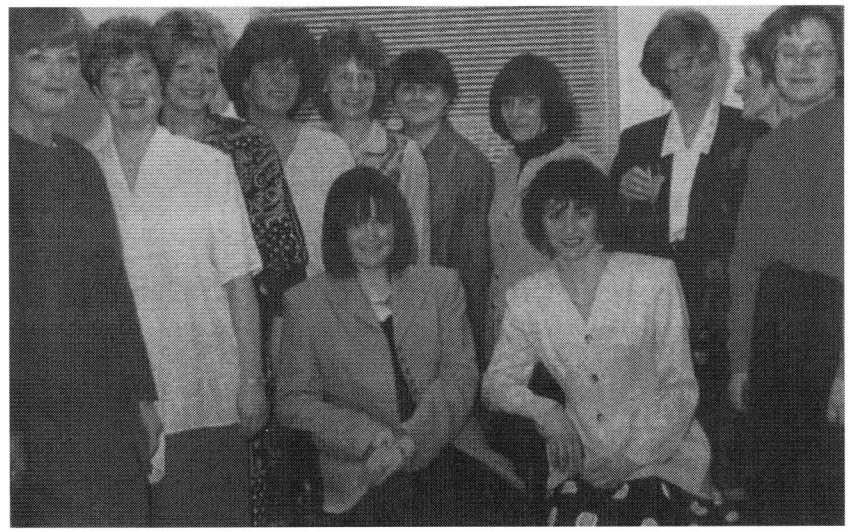

Support staff in 1994
(Charles Hicks Practice archive)

Wives and mothers

Finally, our timeline illustrates the key role played by the wives of the doctors in 19th and early 20th century. They underpinned their medical and business success. Research shows that GP wives in the 1940s provided not only family support and childcare, but often also *'clerical work, tidying the surgery, washing bottles, towels and sheets, paying the bills and dealing with supplies. Some wives ran the infant welfare clinic, while others typed up research work'*.[9] A typical GP practice at that time may have had 'only' 2500 patients, but the workload and commitment required by a spouse, as now, cannot be denied.

Their roles may have changed from the 19th to the 20th century, but we should end by remembering Mercy (Dr Foster), Agnes (Dr Lucas), Grace (Dr Charles Hicks), Lavender (Dr Nelson Hicks) and Cynthia (Dr Rushton) along with all those other wives and female members of their households, many of whose names have not always been recorded. The roles of spouses and partners (male and female) in the 21st century will doubtless be somewhat different, but just as essential. Their stories remain to be written.

Appendix 3

A patient's story: Danny Reid

So, we come to the end of history of the Charles Hicks Practice. It is often said that the age of the 'family doctor' is long gone. That may or may not be true, but Danny's history gives us an unbroken story of using medical practitioners in both Huntingdon and Godmanchester over his lifetime. Danny's story illustrates that the doctors he has encountered have been and remain today in 2024, at the heart of the community.

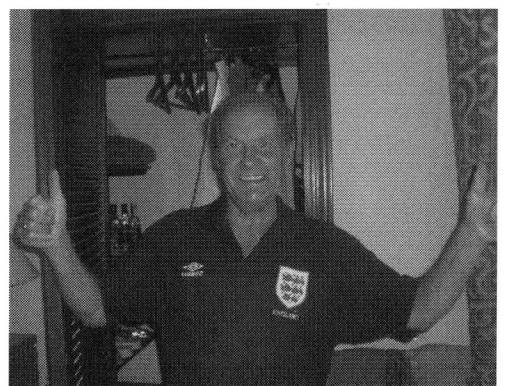
Danny Reid

Danny was born in London in 1936. Evacuated to Huntingdon in 1941 as result of the Blitz, his mother registered Danny and his brother (born in 1939) with Dr Peter Connan's Practice at 84 High Street. Aged seven and with Dr Connan not available Danny was taken to Bosworth House to be seen by Charles Hicks as he needed treatment for 'boils on both knees' that his mother was unable to lance herself. As we have seen, going up some dark stairs to the waiting room with medicine bottles around the walls could be an alarming experience for a child.

Dr Hicks, who is remembered as rather austere and somewhat distant, and referred him to the Town and County Hospital (where both he and Peter Connan worked as medical officers during the war). The hospital doctors treated the boils – but also took the opportunity to keep Danny in hospital and have his tonsils taken out! Although Danny fondly remembers the red dressing gown that the hospital gave him to wear.

Danny's experience shows us the links that continued between the Hicks and Connan Practices. In the 1950s Danny's family were cared for by Peter Connan (notorious locally for his wooden leg), his colleague 'Bunny' Forbes and son 'Dan' Connan. Danny Reid had been at Hinchingbrooke Grammar School with Dan

Connan and so knew him well. Danny's sister was born at home in Bridge Place, Godmanchester in 1943, and the midwife was accompanied by - Charles Hicks.

In 1957 Danny left the Army and returned to Godmanchester but stayed registered with Dr Connan's Practice, which was joined by Dr Derek Cracknell in 1959. Derek Cracknell founded MAGPAS – to which Danny still contributes.

As a Godmanchester resident into the 1960s and 1970s, Danny knew doctors from the Hicks Practice as prominent members of the community. Nelson Hicks is remembered as 'tall and always well-dressed' and 'friends with everyone'. Dr Jim Rushton became a personal friend, and Danny used to visit his house 'out near Gravely' to sample Mrs Rushton's home- made wine.

In the 1980s, for convenience of being more local, Danny registered himself and his family with Dr Gupta in St Anne's Lane. When Dr Gupta retired in 2002, the family transferred to the Hicks Group Practice at Roman Gate.

As patients of over 20 years with the Hicks Group, Danny and his wife have nothing but praise for the treatment that they have received over this time and are 'happy to recommend the Practice to anyone'. They speak of the 'brilliant treatment' from a succession of Roman Gate doctors and nurses now treating Danny for ENT issues and speedily referring him to podiatry and to Hinchingbrooke Hospital for dialysis.

So, even if the 'family doctor' no longer exists the 'community doctors, nurses and other staff at the Hicks Group Practice continue a proud tradition of local treatment.

REFERENCES

Introduction
1. A. Rook, 'General Practice, 1793-1803: The Transactions of a Huntingdonshire Medical Society' (CUP, 2012)

Chapter 1
1. Comparative Account of the Population of Great Britain in the years 1801, 1811, 1821, and 1831. House of Commons (19th October 1831), p118
2. Akeroyd and C. Clifford, 'Huntingdon: Eight Centuries of History' (Breedon Books, 2004), p44
3. K & P. Sneath, 'Godmanchester: A Celebration of 800 Years' (Cambridge: EAH Press, 2011), p64
4. *Ibid.*
5. H.J.M. Green, 'Godmanchester' (Oleander Press, 1977), p45
6. A. Digby, 'The Evolution of British General Practice, 1850 – 1948' (OUP, Oxford, 1999), p201
7. *Ibid.*, p208
8. G.B. Risse, 'Medicine in the Age of Enlightenment' in Medicine in Society: Historical Essays (CUP, 2008), p153
9. S. Gillam, *'Of Patient Bearing – A History of General Practice in Eight* Generations (Hill House Publishing, 2021), p39, 40
10. A. Nicholls, 'Fenland Ague in the Nineteenth Century' in 'Medical History' (CUP 2000), p513-530
11. J. Sutherland and M. Webb, 'So There's Illness In The House: A Brief History of Healthcare in Britain featuring the English Country Town of Towcester' (Kindle edition, 2019)
12. S. Parker, 'A Short History of Medicine', Dorling Kindersley, 2019), p106,107
13. S. Gillam, *op. cit.*, p44
14. S. Gillam, *op. cit.*, p32
15. R. Porter, 'Blood and Guts: A Short History of Medicine' (Penguin, 2003), p34
16. J. Lane, A Social History of Medicine: Health, Healing and Diseases in England, 1750 -1950 (Routledge, 2001), p46
17. S. Gillam, *op. cit.*, p34
18. *Ibid.*
19. A. Rook, 'General Practice, 1793-1803: The Transactions of a Huntingdonshire Medical Society' (CUP, 2012), p240
20. *Ibid.*, p245
21. *Ibid.*, p332
22. A. Digby, *op. cit.*, p150
23. G.B. Risse, *op. cit.*, p180
24. A. Akeroyd and C. Clifford, *op. cit.*, p42
25. R. Carruthers, 'History of Huntingdon: From the Earliest to the Present Times (1824)' (Kessinger Publishing, 2010), p 306
26. A. Rook and M. Carlton, 'The History of Addenbrooke's Hospital, Cambridge', (Cambridge University Press, 1991), p23
27. A. Rook, *op. cit.*, p240
28. G.B. Risse, *op. cit.*, p184

29. A. Digby, *op. cit.*, p237
30. M. Muncaster, 'Medical Services and the Medical Profession in Norfolk: 1815-1911', (Unpublished PhD Thesis, UEA 1976), p50
31. A. Digby, *op. cit.*, p27
32. A. Digby, *op. cit.*, p65

Chapter 2
1. S. Gillam, *'Of Patient Bearing – A History of General Practice in Eight* Generations (Hill House Publishing, 2021), p31
2. G.B. Risse, 'Medicine in the Age of Enlightenment' in Medicine in Society: Historical Essays (CUP, 2008), p130
3. A. Digby, 'Making a Medical Living: Doctors and Patients in the English Market for Medicine, 1720 -1911' (CUP, 1994), p7
4. A. Akeroyd and C. Clifford, 'Huntingdonshire Through Time' (Breedon Publishing, 2004), p41
5. http://www.theprison.org.uk/HuntingdonCB/
6. Provincial Medical & Surgical Journal (1844-1852), Published by BMJ Stable, Vol. 15, No. 21 (Oct. 15, 1851), pp.582-583
7. A. Digby, *op. cit.*, p92
8. A. Digby, *ibid.*
9. A. Digby, *op. cit.*, p107
10. A. Digby *op. cit.*, p28
11. J. Sutherland and M. Webb, 'So There's Illness In The House: A Brief History of Healthcare in Britain featuring the English Country Town of Towcester' (Kindle edition, 2019)
12. Provincial Medical & Surgical Journal, *op. cit.*
13. Ibid.
14. J. Lane, A Social History of Medicine: Health, Healing and Diseases in England, 1750 -1950 (Routledge, 2001), p46
15. R. Carruthers, 'History of Huntingdon: From the Earliest to the Present Times (1824)' (Kessinger Publishing, 2010), p305
16. Ibid.
17. S. Gillam, *op. cit.*, p54
18. A. Digby, *op. cit.*, p241
19. G.B. Risse, *op. cit.*, p180
20. A. Digby, *op. cit.*, p278
21. R. Carruthers, op. cit., p305
22. J. H. Threlfall, 'The Story of Huntingdon County Hospital', (Bluebell Printing, 1978), p5
23. Ibid.
24. S. Parker, A Short History of Medicine', (Dorling Kindersley, 2019), p153-154
25. Dr Nelson Hicks, 'History of Medicine', (Lecture notes in Charles Hicks archive, August 1962), p4
26. J. Lane, *op. cit.*, p140
27. M. Eiloart, 'Huntingdon County Gaol and House of Correction' (Fern House,2009), p32
28. Ibid.
29. Provincial Medical & Surgical Journal, *op. cit.*
30. Dictionary of National Biography,1885-1900, Volume 20. Robert Fox (1798?-1843) by Robert Goodwin
31. A. Rook, *op. cit.*, p 237
32. Huntingdon U3A Local History Group, 'The Huntingdon Institution' (2008), p9

Chapter 3
1. S. Irvine, 'Surgeons and Apothecaries in Suffolk: 1750-1830: City Slickers and Country Bumpkins – Exploring Medical Myths', (Unpublished PhD Thesis, UEA, 2011), p130

2. H.J.M. Green, 'Godmanchester' (Oleander Press, 1977), p45
3. Dr Alex Connan – written testimony (March 2024)
4. J. Lane, A Social History of Medicine: Health, Healing and Diseases in England, 1750 -1950 (Routledge, 2001), p145
5. Dr Nelson Hicks, 'History of Medicine' (Lecture notes in Charles Hicks archive, August 1962), p 4
6. Dr Martin Becker – written testimony (March 2024)
7. J. Lane *op. cit.*, p148
8. Kelly's Directory, 1862
9. M. Eiloart, 'Huntingdon County Gaol and House of Correction' (Fern House,2009)
10. H.J.M. Green, *op. cit.*, p45
11. W. Lee, Report to the General Board of Health, Godmanchester, 1849
12. P. Hornsby, 'Water supplies in Huntingdonshire 1848 -1985' (Pauline Hornsby,1988), p3
13. D. Brunton (ed), 'Medicine Transformed: Health, Disease and Society in Europe 1800-1930' (Open University, 2004), p76
14. J.H. Threlfall, 'The Story of Huntingdon County Hospital', (Bluebell Printing, 1978), p6
15. 'History, Gazetteer & Directory of Huntingdonshire, 1854', p195
16. Kelly's Directory, 1854
17. J. Lane, *op. cit.*, p47
18. J. Lane, *op. cit.*, p164
19. A. Digby, 'Making a Medical Living: Doctors and Patients in the English Market for Medicine, 1720 -1911' (CUP, 1994), p65
20. *Ibid.*, p65
21. Liz Davies (St Neots Museum talk, 2022)
22. C. Lucas, The Fenman's World: Memories of a Fenland Physician (Jarrold and Sons, 1930), p55
23. A. Digby, *op. cit.*, p121
24. History of the Branches of the British medical Association, The British Medical Journal (*Vol. 1, No. 1121 (Jun. 24, 1882)*), pp. 956-959
25. S. Irvine, *op. cit.*, p21
26. A. Digby, *op. cit.*, p132
27. Dr Nelson Hicks, *op. cit.,* p5
28. British Medical Journal, Vol. 1, No. 996 (Jan. 31, 1880), pp. 188-189
29. A. Rook, 'General Practice, 1793-1803: The Transactions of a Huntingdonshire Medical Society' – Part 2' (CUP, 2012), p346-347
30. *Ibid.*, p347
31. Cambridge Community Archives Network, https://www.ccan.co.uk/
32. British Medical Journal, *op. cit.*, pp18

Chapter 4
1. S. Gillam, *'Of Patient Bearing – A History of General Practice in Eight* Generations (Hill House Publishing, 2021), p108
2. A. Digby, 'Making a Medical Living: Doctors and Patients in the English Market for Medicine, 1720 -1911' (CUP, 1994), p127
3. S. Gillam, *op. cit.*, p107
4. A. Akeroyd and C. Clifford, Huntingdon: Eight Centuries of History' (Breedon Books Publishing, 2004), p57
5. J. Lane, A Social History of Medicine: Health, Healing and Diseases in England, 1750 -1950 (Routledge, 2001), p150
6. J. H. Threlfall, 'The Story of Huntingdon County Hospital', (Bluebell Printing, 1978), p9
7. W. Lee, Report to the General Board of Health, Godmanchester, 1849
8. A. Akeroyd and C. Clifford, op. cit., p58

9. https://www.workhouses.org.uk/Huntingdon/Huntingdon1881.shtml
10. https://historicengland.org.uk/research/inclusive-heritage/disability-history/1832-1914/the-changing-face-of-the-workhouse/
11. https://bedsarchives.bedford.gov.uk/Disability/AHistoryOfLocalMentalHealthProvision.aspx - Three Counties Hospital
12. A.S. Monk, 'Three Counties Hospital: A Short History of the Institution 1860 – 1960', p9
13. History of the branches of the British Medical Association (JSTOR)
14. Dr Nelson Hicks, 'History of Medicine' (Lecture notes in the Charles Hicks archive, August 1962), p6
15. J. Sutherland and M. Webb, 'So There's Illness In The House: A Brief History of Healthcare in Britain featuring the English Country Town of Towcester' (Kindle edition, 2019)
16. County Archives, ref RS211/1 – Huntingdon Rural Sanitary Authority Letter Book, 1873-1890
17. S. Gillam op. cit., p105
18. County Archives, ref RS211/2 - Rural Sanitary Authority Minute Book, 1881-1890.
19. County Archives, ref RS211/1, *op. cit.*
20. P. Flower, 'The Life and Times of a Victorian Country Doctor: A Portrait of Reginald Grove. Volume 3 – Life as a Medical Man', (Brown Dog Books, 2022), p477
21. J.H.T. Threlfall, *op. cit.*, p17
22. *Ibid.*, p18
23. County archives, ref 5309/15 – Records of Huntingdon County Hospital
24. D. Brunton (ed), 'Medicine Transformed: Health, Disease and Society in Europe 1800-1930' (Open University, 2004), p167
25. J.H.T Threlfall, *op. cit.,* p18
26. J.H.T Threlfall, *op. cit.,* p21
27. Kelly's Directory, 1914
28. A. Akeroyd and C. Clifford, *op. cit.*, p93
29. Richard Meredith, by personal email, September 2023
30. Kelly's Directory, 1903
31. Kelly's, *op.cit.,*1914
32. Kelly's, *op.cit.,*1914
33. Kelly's, *op.cit.,*1914

Chapter 5
1. Robert Picking on 'History of Huntingdon High Street', Facebook (29th August 2023)
2. P. Flower, 'The Life and Times of a Victorian Country Doctor: A Portrait of Reginald Grove. Volume 3 – Life as a Medical Man', (Brown Dog Books, 2022), p140
3. County Archives, Ref 5309/1 – Charles Hicks (and County Hospital) Confinement Book, 1898 -1945)
4. P. Flower, *op. cit.*, p173
5. P. Flower, *op. cit.*, p 178
6. Kelly's Directory (online), 1903
7. L. Mitton, 'The Victorian Hospital' (Shire Publications, 2008), p29
8. County Archives, Ref 5309/1, *op. cit.*
9. A. Digby, 'Making a Medical Living: Doctors and Patients in the English Market for Medicine, 1720 -1911' (CUP, 1994), p257
10. J. Lane, A Social History of Medicine: Health, Healing and Diseases in England, 1750 -1950 (Routledge, 2001), p79
11. D. Weinbren, 'Bands of Brothers: The roles of friendly Societies in the 19th Century', 2020 (http://www.historyhit.com)
12. Report of the Register of Friendly Societies in England, Appendix to the Report, p 94
13. F.W. Bird, 'Reminiscences of Godmanchester' (Peterborough Advertiser Company, 1911), p 114

References

14. J. Lane, *op. cit.*, p78
15. J. Lane, *op. cit.*, p79
16. S. Gillam, *'Of Patient Bearing – A History of General Practice in Eight* Generations (Hill House Publishing, 2021), p142
17. A. Digby, *op. cit.*, p12
18. A. Digby, *op. cit.*, p307
19. A. Digby, *op. cit.*, p309
20. A. Digby, *op. cit.*, p310
21. J. H. Threlfall, 'The Story of Huntingdon County Hospital', (Bluebell Printing, 1978), p23
22. A. Akeroyd and C. Clifford, 'Huntingdon: Eight Centuries of History' (Breedon Books Publishing, 2004), p66
23. V. Homer, 'Memories from Huntingdon' (Just Print IT, 2000)
24. J.H. Threlfall, *op. cit.*, p23
25. A. Akeroyd and C. Clifford, *op. cit.*, p80
26. J. H. Threlfall, *op. cit.*, p23
27. County Archives, Ref 5309/1 – Charles Hicks (and County Hospital) Confinement Book, 1898-1945
28. R. Leivers and S. Bengree, 'The Godmanchester Bugle: The Great War Journal 1914-1918 (2023)
29. S. Martin, 'A short history of disease' (Pocket Essentials, 2015), p184
30. Dr Martin Becker, Written testimony, (March 2024)
31. S. Martin, *op. cit.*, p 188
32. https://www.visionofbritain.org.uk/unit/10166585/cube/DEATH_TOT
33. Kelly's Directories (library reference), 1914 and 1920
34. A. Akeroyd and C. Clifford, 'Huntingdonshire Through Time' (Amberley Publishing, 2010)
35. A. Digby, 'The Evolution of British General Practice, 1850 – 1948' (OUP, Oxford, 1999), p111-112
36. S. Gillam, *op. cit.*, p142
37. Hunts Post, 21st January 1952, Chares Hicks obituary
38. Dr Nelson Hicks, 'History of Medicine' (Lecture notes in Charles Hicks archive, August 1962), p7
39. Wendy Stukins, Oral testimony, (12th October 2023)
40. Dr Nelson Hicks, *op. cit.*
41. K & P Sneath., 'Thirsty Godmanchester', EAH Press, 2012, p11
42. J. Lane, *op. cit.*, p143
43. https://royalpapworth.nhs.uk/our-hospital/about-us/our-history
44. J. Lane, *op. cit.*, p143
45. Dr Richard Weyell, Written testimony, (March 2024)
46. A. Digby, 'The Evolution of British General Practice', *op. cit.*, p132
47. Dr D Connan and Dr A Connan, Oral testimony, (21st April 2023)
48. A. Digby, 'The Evolution of British General Practice', *op. cit.*, p192
49. S. Gillam, *op. cit.*, p128
50. *Ibid.*, p129
51. *Ibid.*, p141
52. *Ibid.*, p130
53. A. Digby, *op. cit.*, p187-188
54. https://www.nuffieldtrust.org.uk/chapter/inheritance
55. J. H. Threlfall, *op. cit.*, p30
56. Huntingdonshire Cyclist Battalion, http://www.huntscycles.co.uk/Officers/G/Jesse%20Robert%20Garood.htm
57. *Ibid.*, p27
58. *Ibid.*, p29

59. Kelly's Directory (library reference), 1920
60. County Archives, Ref 5309/1, Charles Hicks (and County Hospital) Confinement Book, 1898-1945
61. Census returns, 1939
62. Hinchingbrooke Hospital Record book (1942, (Charles Hicks archive)
63. Dr Alex Connan, Oral testimony, (9th May 2023)
64. John Thackray, Oral testimony, (21st February 2023)
65. Danny Reid, Oral testimony, (19th September 2023)
66. Hunts Post, Funeral notice of Charles Hicks (21st February 1952)
67. David Loose, 'History of Huntingdon High Street', Facebook (August 2023)
68. Hunts Post, *op. cit.*
69. https://awayfromthewesternfront.org/research/soldiers-stories/salonika-medic/

Chapter 6
1. Dr Mike Whitton, Oral testimony, (15th March 2023)
2. *Ibid.*
3. S. Cohen, 'The NHS: Britain's National Health Service, 1948-2020 (Shire Publications, 2020), p13
4. *Ibid.*, p 15-16
5. S. Gillam, *'Of Patient Bearing – A History of General Practice in Eight* Generations (Hill House Publishing, 2021), p159
6. K. Sneath, I Jones et al,' A prescription for Improvement: Towards more rational prescribing in General Practice (London, HMSO 1994)
7. S. Gillam, *op. cit.*, p160
8. S. Gillam, *op. cit.*, p164
9. Robert Picking, 'History of Huntingdon High Street', Facebook, (August 2023)
10. *Ibid.*
11. Pat Roberts, 'History of Huntingdon High Street', Facebook, (September 2023)
12. Dr Nelson Hicks, 'History of Medicine' (lecture notes in Charles Hicks archive, August 1962), p8
13. Dr Mike Whitton, Oral testimony, (15th March 2023)
14. John Thackray, Oral testimony, (21st February 2023)
15. *Ibid.*
16. S. Cohen, 'The District Nurse', (Shire Publications, 2010), p43
17. Verna Hayes, Oral testimony, (7th September 2023)
18. Rita Day, 'Old Codgers and Codgesses of Godmanchester', Facebook (September 2023)
19. Verna Hayes, *op. cit.*
20. Les Williams, Jules Barrell &Tony Dighton, 'Old Codgers and Codgesses of Godmanchester', Facebook (September 2023)
21. Clive Parcell, 'Old Codgers and Codgesses of Godmanchester', Facebook (September 2023)
22. Verna Hayes, *op. cit.*
23. S. Cohen, *op. cit.* p36
24. https://www.encyclopedia.com/social-sciences/culture-magazines/1950s-medicine-and-health-chronology
25. S. Gillam, *op. cit.* p175
26. I. Hardman, 'Fighting for Life', (Viking-Penguin Books, June 2023), p61
27. S. Gillam, *op. cit.* p180
28. Robert Picking, *op. cit.*
29. Dr Alex Connan, Written testimony, (March 2024)
30. Papers relating to the purchase of Bosworth House, Huntingdon, Charles Hicks archive, (passed on by Dr John Stanger in August 2014)

31. Wendy Stukins, Oral testimony, (12th October 2023)
32. S. Gillam, *op. cit.* p180
33. Dr Keith Stewart, Letter to Cambridge Evening News, (13th April 1973)
34. Bill Adams, 'History of Huntingdon High Street', Facebook, (August 2023) –
35. Rosemary Lemmon, 'Old Codgers and Codgesses of Godmanchester', Facebook, (September 2023)
36. John Thackray, *op. cit.*
37. Bill Adams, *op. cit.*
38. Dr Keith Stewart, *op. cit.*

Chapter 7

1. Dr Ian Sweetenham, 'Eulogy for Dr Rushton' (Charles Hicks archive), 6th June 2023
2. Jean Huff, Oral testimony, (12th October 2023)
3. Wendy Stukins, Oral testimony, (12th October 2023)
4. Verna Hayes, Oral testimony, (7th September 2023)
5. S. Gillam, *'Of Patient Bearing – A History of General Practice in Eight* Generations (Hill House Publishing, 2021), p177
6. Wendy Stukins, *op. cit.*
7. Dr Ian Sweetenham, *op. cit.*
8. Cynthia Green, 'Old Codgers and Codgesses of Godmanchester', Facebook, (September 2023)
9. Sneath K & P., 'Godmanchester: A Celebration of 800 Years' (Cambridge: EAH Press, 1911), p192
10. Lesley Wood, Oral testimony, (12th October 2023)
11. MAGPAS, https://magpas.org.uk/our-service/our-history
12. Stephen Gillam, *op. cit.*, p178
13. *Ibid.*, p180
14. *Ibid.*, p186
15. Dr Mike Whitton, Oral testimony, (15th March 2023)
16. Lesley Wood, *op. cit.*
17. Elish Millard, Oral testimony, (January 2004)
18. Lesley Wood, *op. cit.*
19. Dr Mike Whitton, *op. cit.*
20. Sneath K, in 'Records of Huntingdonshire' (Journal of the Huntingdonshire Local History Society, Vol.4 No.5, 2022), p117
21. Hunts Post, Tributes and Messages for Dr Jim Rushton, (11th January 2021)
22. Wendy Stukins, *op. cit.*
23. Lesley Wood, *op. cit.*
24. Stephen Gillam, *op. cit.*, p186
25. *Ibid.*
26. Dr Mike Whitton, *op. cit.*
27. Wendy Stukins, *op. cit.*
28. Dr Mike Whitton, *op. cit.*
29. *Ibid.*
30. Jean Huff, Oral testimony, (12th October 2023)
31. Les Williams, 'Old Codgers and Codgesses of Godmanchester', Facebook, (September 2023)
32. Lesley Wood, *op. cit.*
33. *Ibid.*
34. I. Hardman, 'Fighting for Life', (Viking-Penguin Books, June 2023), p142
35. S. Cohen, 'The NHS: Britain's National Health Service, 1948-2020 (Shire Publications, 2020), p49.
36. I. Hardman, *op. cit.*, p148

37. S. Cohen *op. cit.* p48 and Stephen Gillam, *op. cit.*, p205
38. Dr Mike Whitton, *op. cit.*
39. Dr Martin Becker, Written testimony, (March 2024)
40. *Ibid.*
41. Dr Ian Sweetenham, *op. cit.*

Chapter 8
1. Dr Ian Sweetenham, Oral testimony, (February 2024)
2. S. Gillam, *'Of Patient Bearing – A History of General Practice in Eight* Generations (Hill House Publishing, 2021) p 208
3. Lesley Wood, Oral testimony, (12th October 2023)
4. Wendy Stukins, Oral testimony, (12th October 2023)
5. Gillam, *op. cit.*, p212
6. Dr Ian Sweetenham, *op. cit.*
7. S. Gillam, *op. cit.*, p211
8. https://www.nuffieldtrust.org.uk/chapter/1988-1997-new-influences-and-new-pathways
9. Dr Mike Whitton, Oral testimony, (15th March 2023)
10. I. Hardman, 'Fighting for Life', (Viking-Penguin Books, June 2023), p201
11. *Ibid.*, p154
12. *Ibid.*, p219
13. Dr Ian Sweetenham, *op. cit.*
14. Dr Ian Sweetenham, *op. cit.*
15. S. Gillam, *op. cit.*, p215
16. I. Hardman, *op. cit.*, p219
17. Dr Mike Whitton, *op. cit.*
18. S. Gillam, *op. cit.*, p202
19. I. Hardman, *op. cit.*, p202
20. S. Cohen, 'The NHS: Britain's National Health Service, 1948-2020 (Shire Publications, 2020), p53
21. *Ibid.*, p54
22. S. Gillam, *op. cit.*, p221
23. *Ibid.*, p217
24. *Ibid.*, p218
25. Dr Mike Whitton, *op. cit.*
26. PULSE Health Journal, (25th March 2014)
27. S. Gillam, op. cit., p218,219
28. Hicks group Practice Quality Report (2016), https://api.cqc.org.uk/public/v1/reports/dcb36d33-16c4-4fa8-be12-f1dbea53c268?20210123061046
29. Dr Ian Sweetenham, Written testimony, (3rd March 2024)
30. Irena Hall, Oral testimony, (5th March 2024)
31. GP patient workload and GP numbers, https://rcgp.org.uk
32. P. Hewitt, 'The Hewitt Review of Integrated Care Systems', April 2023
33. https://www.kingsfund.org.uk/audio-video/key-facts-figures-nhs
34. GP patient workload and GP numbers, https://rcgp.org.uk
35. I*bid.*, GP experiences from tracking survey of 1262 GPs in 2022
36. Irena Hall, *op. cit.*
37. Dr Carolyn Smithson, Written testimony, (7th March 2024)

Appendix 2
1. Provincial Medical and Surgical Journal, Jonah Wilson, (1844-1852) Vol 15, No.21, Oct.15, 1851, pp 584-585

References

2. S. Gillam, *'Of Patient Bearing – A History of General Practice in Eight* Generations (Hill House Publishing, 2021), p34
3. J. H. Threlfall, 'The Story of Huntingdon County Hospital', (Bluebell Printing, 1978), p22
4. A. Digby, 'The Evolution of British General Practice, 1850 – 1948' (OUP, Oxford, 1999), p292
5. J.H. Threlfall, *op. cit.*
6. L. Jefferson & K. Bloor, 'Women in Medicine: historical perspectives and recent trends', British Medical Bulletin, June 2015
7. Number of registered doctors in the UK in 2024, https://digital.nhs.uk/data-and-information/publications/statistical/general-and-personal-medical-services/29-february-2024
8. PULSE Health Journal, (25th March 2014)
9. Women in general practice: The family unit', Royal College of General Practitioners, https://www.rcgp.org.uk/about/museum-heritage/women-gp-exhibition

Index of Names

Adams, Bill 63, 64
Allbutt, Thomas, Dr. 22, 88
Allvey, Samuel, Dr. 8
Armitage, Miss 34, 42, 91

Baker, Jackie 71
Baker, Lorraine 83, 93
Ballard, Janice 82
Barrell, Jules 60
Barriman, Miss 33, 34
Baumgartner, John, Dr. 14, 22
Beart, Agnes 28, 31, 35, 39, 94
Beart, Robert 29
Becker, Martin, Dr. 74
Bevan, Nye 56
Bulstrode, Sean, Dr. 85, 90

Cairns, Harry 72
Carver, Edmund, Dr. 26
Cattle, Valerie 71
Chadwick, Edwin 18, 87
Collings, Joseph 57, 89
Connan, Anne, Dr. 47, 50, 51, 62, 92
Connan, Dan, Dr. 62, 72, 73, 95, 96
Connan, Peter, Dr. 47-52, 54, 60, 62, 72, 95
Cooper, Astley, Sir 11, 12
Cooper, Mercy 17, 25, 95
Cracknell, Derek, Dr. 62, 67, 72, 96
Crawford, Miss 33

Davis, William, Morriston 24
Day, Rita 60
Densem, Sophie, Dr. 81, 90, 92
Desborough, Mr. 8, 11, 12
Dickson, Zoe 83
Dighton, Tom 77
Dighton, Tony 60
Duckitt, Irene 71

Evans, Gail 71
Falla, Ernest, Dr. 62

Ferrelly, Sandy 82
Forbes, Bunny, Dr. 62, 95
Foster, Michael (Jnr) 17, 25, 26
Foster, Michael (Snr), Dr. 4, 12, 15 -17, 19 -27, 29, 44, 76, 87, 93
Fox, Martyn 87
Fox, Pat 82, 87
Fox, Robert, Dr. 8, 14, 16, 52
France, Dr. 66, 87
Frank, Johann 18

Garrood, Jesse, Robert, Dr. 25, 50, 53
George, Lloyd 39, 70, 79
Grady, Laura, Dr. 85
Gray, Sharon 72
Green, Cynthia 66
Green, Michael 1, 19
Greenwood, Arthur, Dr. 50, 51, 54
Grove, Reginald, Dr. 38
Gupta, Dr. 61, 71, 80, 96

Hall, Irena 84
Halstead, William 34, 88
Harrison, Lisa 83, 93
Hayes, Verna 59 - 61, 66
Herbert, Lucas, Dr. 4, 15, 19, 24, 27, 28, 31- 36, 39, 41, 43, 44, 48, 88
Hicks, Charles, Dr. 3, 4, 8, 27, 35 - 55, 59 - 61, 68, 88, 93, 95, 96
Hicks, Grace 39, 49, 51, 94
Hicks, Lavender 53, 55, 57, 58, 64, 94
Hicks, Nelson, Dr. 1, 14, 18, 24, 27, 31, 39, 45, 48, 51, 53 - 65, 67, 76, 89, 93, 96
Hoffman, Felix 43
Huff, Jean 72
Hynes, Dr. 54, 60, 64, 68

Isaacson, Wotton, Dr. 22, 24, 26

Jackson, Jamie, Dr. 85
James, Anne 82

Jenner, Edward 14, 87
Jones, Pat 82

Keen, Richard 11
Koch, Robert 34, 88

Laennec, Rene 13, 87
Laxton, Sue 71
Lee, William 19, 20
Lemmon, Rosemary 64
Lister, Joseph 34, 88
Liston, Robert 21, 87
Love, William, Dr 62, 67

Manning, Anne 10
Mart, Doreen 59 - 61, 66, 91
May, Eileen 63, 66
McRitchie, David, Dr. 32, 33, 36, 39
McRitchie, Donald, Dr. 32, 33, 36, 39, 47
Middlemiss, John, Dr. 61, 66, 67, 71
Middlemiss, Maggie 82
Milburn, Alan 79
Millard, Betty 71
Millard, Elish 68, 82
Montague, Mary, Lady 14
Morton, Dr. 13
Moseley, Karen 83

Nightingale, Florence 33, 34, 88

Olufemi, Taiwo, Dr. 85

Parcell, Clive 60
Peck, Mr 17
Phillips, Dr. 62
Platten, Harriet, Dr. 78, 89, 92
Powell, Baden 39
Powell, Enoch 61
Pritchard, Martin, Dr. 62

Raemdonck, Heinz, Van, Dr. 80
Reid, Danny 52, 95
Robert, Picking 58, 62
Roberts, Pat 58
Rushton, Cynthia 66, 75, 94
Rushton, Jim, Dr. 4, 62 - 66, 68 - 76, 78, 89, 93, 96
Rust, James 9, 22

Saunders, Florence 42
Semmelweis, Ignaz 31, 87

Sibthorpe, Dr. 62
Simpson, James 21, 87
Slade, Joshua 35
Smithson, Carolyn, Dr. 81, 86, 89, 92, 93
Smith, William 11, 16
Snow, John, Dr. 18, 87
Soni, Urjit, Dr. 81, 90
Springthorpe, Emily 51
Stanger, Dr. 72, 78, 80, 84, 89
Stewart, Keith, Dr. 63 - 65, 68, 72, 74, 75, 78, 89
Stukins, Wendy 63, 68 -70, 72, 79
Sweetenham, Ian, Dr. 72 - 75, 78, 80, 81, 84, 89

Tester, Mary 36, 51
Thackray, John 52, 59, 64, 82
Turnill, Adelaide, Dr. 68, 78, 89, 91

Varrier-Jones, Pendrill 46
Veitch, Dr 50, 51
Venkat-Raman, Akhila, Dr 85

Ward, William, Dr. 14, 16, 21, 22, 24, 26
Wass, Mr 11
Weyell, Richard, Dr. 75, 78, 79, 89
Whitton, Mike, Dr. 55, 70 - 73, 78, 82, 89
Williams, Les 60, 67, 71
Wilson, Jonah 3, 4, 11-13, 15 -17, 19, 20, 82, 87, 91
Wilson, Pat 82
Wood, Alexander 24, 88
Wood, Lesley 67, 68, 70, 72, 79
Wu, Edward, Dr. 85, 90

GENERAL INDEX

Acorn Surgery 80, 89
Addenbrooke's Hospital 9, 26, 42, 79, 87
Additional Roles Reimbursement Scheme (ARRS) 85
Ague 6, 15, 23, 25
AIDS 73, 89
Amputations 7, 12, 13
Anaesthetic 7, 12, 20, 21, 50, 87
Anatomy Act (1832) 10, 11, 87
Antenatal 79
Antibiotics 46, 61
Antiseptic 31, 88
Apothecaries Act (1815) 12, 87
Apothecary 7, 11, 12, 16, 17, 20, 26, 27
Aspirin 43
Asthma 10, 79

Benefit Clubs 40
Beveridge Report (1942) 88
Bloodletting 6, 7, 13, 25
Board of Health 19, 20, 32
Bosworth House 35 - 37, 39, 42, 44, 47, 51 - 59, 61 - 63, 65, 88, 95
British Medical Association (BMA) 23, 31, 56, 88
Bronchitis 48, 58

Care Quality Commission (CQC) 81, 83, 90
Cataract 8
Chicken pox 6, 48
Cholera 1, 16, 17, 18, 19, 34, 87
Cholesterol 67
Community Care Act (1990) 73, 89
County Gaol 11, 15, 23, 29, 34, 35
COVID 1, 3, 43, 75, 84, 90

Daffy's Elixir 23
Dermatology 79, 81
Diabetes 61, 67, 79, 80, 81
Diphtheria 31, 48, 61
Dispensary 8, 9, 13, 14, 15, 16, 22, 87

District Nurse 59, 60
Elixir 23
Ermine Street Surgery 66, 74, 77, 89

Factory Surgeon 21, 27, 44
Family Doctor Charter (1965) 63, 89
Family Planning 67
Fitzwilliam Hunt 55
Forceps 7, 31
Friendly Society 27, 40
Fund Holding 79, 89

General Medical Council (GMC) 21, 88
Godfrey's Cordial 7, 23
Guy's Hospital 11, 27, 37, 38, 54, 55, 68

Health and Care Act (2022) 85, 90
Health and Social Care Act (2012) 81, 90
Hinchingbrooke Hospital 70, 73, 74, 89, 96
Home Births 31, 39, 50, 59, 60, 91
Humours 6
Huntingdonshire Medical Society 4, 8, 16, 17, 76, 87
Huntingdon Town and County Hospital 87
Hypodermic syringe 24

Influenza 30, 48
Innominate Club 55
Inoculation 14

Lancet, the 10, 57, 87
Laudanum 6, 13, 23
Leeches 6, 13, 18

MAGPAS 62, 67, 72, 89, 96
Measles 6, 48, 58, 61
Medical Officer of Health 16, 32, 36, 44, 46, 47, 50
Medico-Chirurgical Society 16, 25
Miasma 6, 18
Microscope 49, 50

Midwife 7, 36, 59, 60, 68, 88, 91, 96
Midwives Act (1902) 39, 88
Midwives Act (1936) 50, 88
Ministry of Health 43, 46
Multi-Disciplinary Team (MDT) 85
Mumps 48

National Health Service Act (1946) 56, 57, 59, 61, 63
National Insurance Act (1911) 39, 40, 46, 88
Norris Museum 20, 21, 24, 76

Obesity 67
Old Court Hall 3, 66, 69 - 72, 77, 89
Ophthalmoscope 21
Opiates 6
Opium powder 13

Panel Doctor 39, 40, 41, 45
Papworth Village Settlement 46, 88
Parkinson's Disease 25
Patients' Forum 1, 68, 82, 83, 90
Penicillin 48, 61, 88
Pest House 18, 34, 35
Petersfield Hospital 19, 56, 66, 88
Pharmacy 12
Physician 5, 7, 8, 13, 14, 22, 24, 27, 91
Pneumonia 28, 31, 43, 48
Polio 61
Poor Law Medical Officer 21
Post Office 44
Primary Care Act (1997) 89
Primrose Lane Hospital 62
Priory Fields Surgery 72, 73
Public Health Act (1848) 19, 87
Public Health Act (1875) 29, 32, 88
Public Vaccinator 15, 32, 36, 44, 50

Quacks 10, 22, 23
Quality Outcomes Framework (QOF) 80, 83, 89
Quinine 13, 25, 43

RAF Wyton 65, 66, 69, 89
Red Cross 42, 43, 54, 91
Rheumatology 78, 79
Roman Gate Surgery 3, 4, 11, 59, 69, 77, 78, 80, 81, 84, 89, 90
Royal College of Physicians (RCP) 14, 36, 55, 65
Royal College of Surgeons (RCS) 16, 21, 27, 28, 36, 38, 55, 65

Scarlet Fever 6, 48
Scurvy 10, 15
Septicemia 32
Smallpox 1, 6, 10, 14 -16, 18, 23, 30, 34, 37, 61, 87
Smallpox Vaccination Act (1853) 87
Spanish Flu 1, 25, 43
Steroids 61
Stethoscope 12, 13, 49, 59, 87
Strychnine 24, 31
St Thomas' Hospital 33, 34
Surgeon 6, 7, 8, 11, 12, 15 - 17, 19 - 22, 25 - 29, 32, 36, 39, 41, 42, 44, 47, 50, 51, 91, 92
Syphilis 8, 28, 88

Thermometer 22, 88
Three Counties Hospital 30, 88
Transactions 4, 8, 16, 17, 21, 36, 53, 76
Tuberculosis 13, 28, 46, 48, 52, 61, 88
Typhoid 6, 19, 48
Typhus 6, 8, 29, 30

University College Hospital 17

Vaccination 14, 15, 57, 60, 61, 75, 84, 87

Walden House 42, 43, 88, 91
Walnut Tree House 19, 52, 88
Whooping Cough 48, 61
Workhouse 3, 19, 20, 23, 27, 29, 30, 32, 39, 52, 87, 88
World War One (WW1) 36, 42, 43, 47, 50, 54, 91
World War Two (WW2) 51, 92

X-ray 50, 54, 70